HOW TO COPE
SUCCESSFULLY WITH THE

IRRITABLE BOWEL DIET

RICHARD EMERSON

Wellhouse Publishing Ltd

First published in Great Britain in 2005 by
Wellhouse Publishing Ltd
31 Middle Bourne Lane
Lower Bourne
Farnham, Surrey GU10 3NH

DISCLAIMER

The aim of this book is to provide general information only and should
not be treated as a substitute for the medical advice of your doctor or
any other health care professional. The publisher and author is not
responsible or liable for any diagnosis made by a reader based on the
contents of this book. Always consult your doctor if you are in any way
concerned about your health.

A catalogue record for this book is available from the British Library

ISBN 10 digit: 1 903784 19 0
ISBN 13 digit: 978 1 903784 19 8

Also by Richard Emerson in the How to Cope Successfully series:
   Irritable Bowel Syndrome

Printed and bound in Great Britain by
Creative Print & Design Group, Middlesex UB7 0LW

To Elsie-Louisa Emerson for her love,
support and encouragement

Acknowledgements

The author would like to thank Dr Natasha Bye, Scientific Affairs, Nutricia Limited; Sue McGarrigle, Technical Advisor, BioCare Ltd; and my editor Solveig Gardner Servian for their valuable help and advice, and Asda Stores Ltd, BioCare Ltd, Duncan Baird Publishers Ltd, Marshall Cavendish Ltd and Yakult UK Ltd, for permission to use their recipes. Leek and Potato Soup, and Artichoke Hearts, Broad Beans and Shiitake Mushrooms copyright © Duncan Baird Publishers Ltd. Braised Chicory copyright © and courtesy of Marshall Cavendish Ltd.

Contents

About the author

Richard Emerson is a specialist health writer and editor with over 25 years' publishing experience. He is a member of the UK Medical Journalists' Association and has contributed to a broad range of health reference and self-help books including: *The Stress Factor, You & Your Heart, Get Fit Feel Fantastic, The Best Sex You'll Ever Have*. Having written How To Cope Successfully With *Irritable Bowel Syndrome* for Wellhouse Publishing (published in 2002) Richard felt that a specific IBS Diet book would add considerably to the advice given in the previous book. Richard lives and works in Berkshire.

Introduction

This is the second book I have written on IBS. The first, *How to Cope Successfully with Irritable Bowel Syndrome*, looks at all the studies that have been carried out into the causes and treatment of this condition. It includes a section on diet, as well as chapters on pain management, stress, medication and much more besides.

At the time it was written, research was revealing fascinating insights into the role of the nerves and nerve receptors that control the digestive tract. Drug companies had high hopes that this knowledge would give rise to a new generation of 'magic bullets' – a range of problem-free pills that would bring IBS symptoms under control. Indeed some drugs have undergone clinical trials. But the longed-for drug breakthrough has failed to materialize (so far), and IBS continues to need a multi-targeted approach: diet, stress management and other lifestyle changes, along with medication as required.

In the last two years, the most promising field of research to impact on IBS has been in microbiology. As the mysterious microflora of the gut have revealed more of their secrets to researchers, two new terms have entered the language – 'probiotics' and 'prebiotics'. They refer to the bacterial guardians of the digestive tract that keep us from harm, and the special food they need to thrive. They play such an important part in the management of IBS that they deserve their own chapter. In recent years, more has been discovered about the fruits, vegetables, herbs and spices that are of particular benefit in IBS. They, too, require more space to be devoted to them. All in all it seemed like a good time to write a book looking at IBS and diet in some detail. So here it is. Bon Appetit!

Chapter One

Symptoms and Causes of IBS

Irritable bowel syndrome (IBS) is a common problem that is, at best, unpleasant and inconvenient, and at worst highly distressing and debilitating. In many cases the condition can blight a person's life.

There may be many people today who suffer from this condition without realizing it, or seeking the advice of a doctor. They simply soldier on, relying on over-the-counter remedies to help them cope with their symptoms. It is often only in the more debilitating cases that sufferers seek medical help. So it is impossible to know the full extent of the problem. Even so, IBS is the most common condition treated by gastroenterologists, the doctors who specialize in disorders of the digestive tract.

Doctors can offer a range of drugs to alleviate the symptoms of IBS. But whether taken on prescription or over the counter, medication is only part of the solution. This is because symptoms tend to recur unless sufferers make the all-important dietary and other lifestyle changes that will truly make a difference to their quality of life.

This book will focus mainly on those dietary measures, although other lifestyle changes are discussed briefly later in the book. For a more comprehensive look at IBS as a whole, see the companion book to this one called *How to Cope Successfully with Irritable Bowel Syndrome (Wellhouse Publishing)*.

What is the Bowel?

The bowel (also known as the intestines, or 'gut') is the long, muscular tube that runs from the stomach to the anus. It forms the main part of the gastrointestinal (GI) tract and is divided up into the small bowel (small intestine) and the large bowel (large intestine). The bowel – and the rest of the GI tract – performs many important tasks. For example, it produces the various enzymes, stomach acids and bile salts needed to break down lumps of food into particles tiny enough to pass through the gut lining.

The bowel must be able to absorb – and, in some cases, manufacture – all the vitamins and minerals needed for health. It must take in enough water to satisfy our physical needs and prevent dehydration, but not so much that we become constipated.

The bowel is also an important defensive barrier, helping to neutralize toxic substances in the food and produce antibodies and immune system cells to combat infection. Last, and by no means least, it must pass waste matter out of the body.

What is Irritable Bowel Syndrome?

The term 'irritable bowel syndrome' covers a wide range of symptoms, but all are related to problems involving the bowel. The term 'irritable', in this context, means that the bowel is hypersensitive. It reacts in an extreme way to particular foods and drinks that in other people cause no symptoms at all. This hypersensitivity is often linked to hormonal changes, such as those occurring just before menstruation, or emotional upsets, tension or chronic stress. IBS symptoms tend to be worst when several factors combine.

'Syndrome' means the condition produces wide-ranging symptoms. All individuals are unique, so no two IBS sufferers will experience the same pattern of symptoms. What's more, the pattern of symptoms may change from time to time – month by month, week by week or even daily. Symptoms can get worse, improve or disappear for a while before returning. And so the cycle repeats.

Some symptoms are experienced by most sufferers. These include bowel problems: diarrhoea and/or constipation, abdominal pain, bloating and flatulence. But there are other symptoms, such as nausea, dyspepsia, excess urination and even back pain, that are more common with IBS, although not all sufferers will experience them.

Bowel Symptoms

Typically, IBS sufferers have a problem with their bowel habit – that is, how often they visit the lavatory. They feel they need to go either too often or not often enough. Some find they have to visit the lavatory at frequent intervals throughout the day. This is called diarrhoea-dependent IBS (D-IBS). Even more upsetting than the frequency is that the urge to go may come on rapidly and urgently, often at the most inappropriate times. Sufferers may fear they won't reach a lavatory in time. Even if this feeling only happens occasionally, the sense of urgency and fear of embarrassment can destroy a person's confidence and severely restrict their freedom of movement, sometimes making them virtual prisoners in their own homes.

At the other end of the scale, some sufferers only get the urge to visit the lavatory a few times a week, or else go to the bathroom regularly but never feel they have finished. This is called constipation-dependent IBS (C-IBS), and this, too, can be distressing. Although C-IBS may not be as restricting as D-IBS, sufferers can become obsessed with their bowel habit, causing stress, anxiety and depression.

Sometimes IBS symptoms swing from one extreme to the other, starting with periods of constipation, followed by a brief period of normality, before entering the diarrhoea-dependent stage. This is known as alternating IBS (A-IBS).

Pain and Wind

Along with an irregular bowel habit, IBS sufferers typically experience abdominal pain. The extent and form of this pain varies from person to person, but may be sharp, burning, aching or colicky (coming and going). It may be felt in one part of the abdomen, or more generally over a wider area. For some sufferers, the pain is so severe they have to lie down until it passes.

Another common symptom is wind – a build-up of intestinal gas, causing bloating, and potentially embarrassing burping and flatulence. This may start as soon as you awake in the morning. IBS sufferers may have a relatively flat stomach at first. But the gas builds up steadily throughout the day, giving a distended appearance to the abdomen that women often say makes them look pregnant. This build-up of gas pressure can cause abdominal pain, sometimes only relieved by breaking wind.

Rumbling and Other Symptoms

Even non-sufferers find their stomach 'rumbles' from time to time, especially when they are hungry. But it is much more common, and more extreme, in IBS. It is usually heard as a loud gurgling, caused by the gut contents shuffling back and forth. This is yet another potential source of embarrassment. IBS sufferers frequently report a wide range of other symptoms, including nausea, poor appetite or premature satiety (feeling full before you have finished a normal-size meal), heartburn, depression and fatigue, among many others.

Warning Signs

One point to stress is that IBS, while distressing, is not life-threatening. Nor is it as debilitating as disorders such as inflammatory bowel disease (IBD), Crohn's disease, or ulcerative colitis. However, many of these conditions have similar symptoms. So it is vitally important to recognize any symptoms that are not associated with IBS but that might indicate a serious underlying disorder. These are called 'red flag' symptoms and require an urgent visit to your doctor. They include:

- bleeding from the anus or blood on the stools (this can also be a sign of haemorrhoids, or 'piles', which, although not so serious, is a painful condition requiring treatment)

- unexplained weight loss (that is, losing weight even though you are eating normally and are not more active than normal)
- persistent abdominal pain (especially if it wakes you up at night)
- abdominal bloating that persists overnight
- unexplained vomiting
- food that sticks in the throat
- unexplained breathlessness
- abnormal swelling
- unexplained rash

What Causes IBS?

Although much of the condition remains a mystery, a general understanding of the condition is slowly emerging. IBS is called a 'functional' gut disorder, meaning that the problem relates to the way the bowel normally operates. The problem involves a network of nerves called the enteric nervous system that controls the digestive tract. The enteric system is linked to autonomic nerve pathways (sympathetic and parasympathetic nervous systems) that control other automatic functions such as heart rate and blood flow. The enteric system is also influenced indirectly by sensory nerves that inform the brain about painful stimuli in the bowel.

There is some evidence to show that there is an inherited weakness in IBS sufferers. This may not reveal itself unless triggered by factors such as food poisoning or antibiotic treatment. The more trigger factors there are, the more likely the person is to suffer from IBS.

As a result, nerve pathways between the gut and the brain become hypersensitive, reacting in an extreme and unpredictable way to stimuli – such as rich or spicy foods, citrus fruit, coffee, dairy foods, wheat – that cause no reaction in others. These stimuli most often cause symptoms at times of tension, anxiety or stress, for example, when under work or exam pressure, or following emotional upset, or prior to menstruation.

Microbes and Trauma

The most common trigger for IBS is gut infection, often contracted on holiday. Many sufferers pinpoint the start of their problems to a 'tummy bug' and say they have 'never really felt right since'. As well as causing hypersensitivity, infection upsets the delicate microfloral balance in the gut, in which beneficial bacteria prevent the spread of harmful (pathogenic) organisms. A course of antibiotics can also trigger IBS, because the beneficial bacteria are destroyed along with the harmful ones, but take longer to recover.

Major surgery, especially involving the bowel and/or lower abdomen, is another important factor linked to IBS. In part, this may again be due to the antibiotics often given routinely as a preventive measure against post-operative infection. The role of beneficial bacteria in gut health is covered in Chapter Three.

Most people recover from food poisoning without further problems. But for IBS sufferers, symptoms can continue long after the original illness has passed. Infection causes inflammation, which over-stimulates the sensory receptors in the bowel. Inflammation also hypersensitizes the nerve pathways between the bowel and brain. Repeat infection increases this sensitivity, so exacerbating symptoms.

If IBS symptoms arise directly from gastrointestinal infection, the condition is called post-infectious IBS (P-IBS). P-IBS is associated with amoebic, bacterial, fungal and viral infection (especially *Campylobacter* and candida).

There are other changes identified in the bowel of patients with P-IBS that are not seen in healthy subjects, for example changes in the levels of signalling chemicals such as serotonin, and increased permeability or 'leakiness' (see below).

IBS is also linked to emotional and physical trauma such as severe injury, violent crime (especially rape), bereavement, a problem home environment, and time in institutional care, such as a children's home, the armed services or prison.

Leaky Gut Syndrome
Severe gastrointestinal infection can cause a condition called leaky gut syndrome (LGS). Although common, this condition is poorly recognized and rarely investigated. LGS follows acute inflammation or damage to the bowel, causing large spaces to open up in the mucous lining. Normally, only tiny food particles can cross the gut wall. A leaky gut, however, allows infectious organisms and the toxins they produce to bypass this barrier and release toxins into the gut that disrupt normal bowel function. The flood of toxins can also overburden the liver, inhibiting its ability to deal effectively with everyday chemicals, and can cause wide-ranging health effects, such as arthritis.

Leaky gut syndrome is also associated with fibromyalgia, a mysterious condition featuring widespread chronic pain, fatigue and stiffness, sleep disturbances, anxiety and depression. Around 60 per cent of fibromyalgia patients also have IBS, 80 per cent also have chronic fatigue syndrome and 33 per cent have multiple chemical sensitivity – a severe adverse reaction to common household chemicals.

A leaky gut also allows through food particles that are larger than the immune system will tolerate. The bowel then reacts against food substances previously regarded as harmless, leading to food intolerance and allergy. Once the gut wall is damaged, transport mechanisms that carry vital minerals, such as magnesium and copper, become disrupted, causing deficiency symptoms.

Whether leaky gut syndrome is a cause of IBS or a separate illness in its own right is questionable, but LGS symptoms, such as alternating diarrhoea and constipation, abdominal pain, excess wind and bloating, seem to mirror those seen in IBS.

The Outlook for IBS

There is no 'cure' as such for IBS, but this doesn't mean that the outlook is one of despair. Most chronic sufferers learn to manage IBS through a combination of lifestyle changes (see Chapter Eleven), over-the-counter remedies and, if appropriate, prescription drugs. By managing the condition they lessen their symptoms to the extent that IBS causes minimal disruption to their lives. They no longer feel preoccupied with – or dominated by – the condition and so lead full, active, 'normal' lives.

Even better news. In some cases the condition clears up of its own accord, often relatively quickly. In the 1990s, German researchers followed up a group of hospital patients who had received treatment for IBS some ten years previously. Less than 10 per cent had continuing symptoms and 20 per cent had forgotten they ever had IBS!

Tackling IBS
The best approach is to manage your symptoms through diet and other lifestyle changes. An important preliminary step is to look at how your diet can be improved. First, you must identify and avoid (or limit) foods that trigger symptoms, or that make them worse. Second, you must eat more of the foods that ease or eliminate symptoms.

A vital food component often missing in the modern diet is fibre. For IBS sufferers, getting the right fibre balance is critical. Digestive upsets can be caused by too little fibre or even too much. Including the right level and type of fibre in the diet helps reduce or prevent IBS symptoms, and provides many other important health benefits. Friendly bacteria have a vital role to play in a healthy diet, too. All these aspects of IBS management are discussed in the following chapters.

Chapter Two

Avoiding Problem Foods

The exact role foods play in IBS is unclear – and widely disputed by researchers. Some experts claim that one of the underlying causes is likely to be allergy or intolerance to a food. If so, the sufferer will normally react each time that food is eaten.

A few studies have shown a direct link between food intolerance and IBS in a few people, but these represent only a tiny percentage of total sufferers. This has led some researchers to dispute the claim that food intolerance plays a significant role in IBS. However, others say that you need to regularly eat at least 100 g (4 oz) of a problem food before symptoms develop, and that test foods used in scientific trials fall short of this.

An IBS sufferer's adverse reaction to certain foods could indicate a 'sensitivity', rather than intolerance. In IBS, the nerves that control the bowel become hypersensitive at times of emotional upset or stress. So any food that triggers a strong response in the sensory receptors that 'report' on chemical conditions in the gut (chemoreceptors) can trigger an exaggerated response in IBS sufferers, leading to symptoms.

Food Allergy

A food allergy is an extreme reaction by the immune system to something you've eaten. At times of heightened immune system activity (following a severe infection, for example), certain components in a food may be falsely identified as a threat. Often they have a similar molecular profile to some component in the organism the immune system is fighting. In other cases the problem may stem from a disorder called leaky gut syndrome (see Chapter One). This causes the gut wall to become excessively porous, or 'leaky', and allow through larger food molecules than the immune system is used to dealing with. This, too, can cause an allergic reaction.

Most foods have the potential to cause an allergy. Common causes of allergy (allergens) include nuts, fish, shellfish, eggs, chocolate, berries, milk and additives, such as colourings and preservatives. Two foods that rarely if ever provoke a reaction, however, are lamb and pears.

There are several tests for food allergies. For sufferers, there are two solutions: avoid the food or undergo a course of desensitizing treatment (see Chapter Twelve).

Food intolerance is due to an inability to tolerate or break down and absorb certain foods. This condition is sometimes called 'false food allergy', because symptoms can be similar (and often more severe) than true allergy. The mechanisms involved, however, although poorly understood, are different. The two principal causes of food intolerance are gluten (found in wheat and other cereals) and lactose (found in dairy products).

Gluten and Coeliac Disease

Gluten is a protein found in many cereals, including wheat. In some people, the presence of gluten triggers an extreme 'auto-immune' response in which the immune system attacks the lining of the small intestine, causing inflammation and damage. This condition, called coeliac disease, can cause IBS-like symptoms, such as excess gas, bloating and diarrhoea. In some cases the condition inhibits absorption of other nutrients, causing malnutrition and weight loss. Unlike IBS, there are tests that can be carried out to identify coeliac disease (see Chapter Twelve).

IBS is not connected with coeliac disease as such. They are different disorders. But a mild sensitivity to gluten may trigger IBS symptoms in some people. Many sufferers find that by avoiding or cutting down on wheat products they can reduce the frequency and severity of symptoms. There are many types of wholegrains available that make healthy alternatives to wheat and yet do not trigger IBS symptoms (see Chapter Seven).

Wheat flour is used in a wide range of products. As well as bread, pastries, biscuits and cakes, it is used in batter and breadcrumb coatings, packet soups and sausages, and as a thickening in casseroles and stews. If you think gluten may trigger symptoms, many shops sell gluten-free wheat, pasta, biscuits, flour and other products.

Milk and Lactose Intolerance

Lactose is the principal sugar in milk. Those who lack the enzyme lactase, needed to digest this sugar, suffer lactose intolerance. As a consequence, lactose passes through the digestive tract in undigested form until it reaches the bowel. Here it is broken down by pathogenic gut bacteria, causing IBS-like symptoms such as abdominal pain, bloating, flatulence and diarrhoea.

The fact that many human adults (mainly of Indo-European origin) can digest milk is something of a quirk of nature. Most mammals lose this ability once they are weaned. Even among humans, lactose intolerance is the norm rather than the exception, affecting around three-quarters of the adult population worldwide.

If you decide to eliminate from your diet all products containing milk, you will have to take care when buying processed foods such as biscuits, cakes, puddings, sauces and many ready meals, which often contain milk ingredients. These may be listed on food labels, with or without their E numbers (see Chapter Five) as lactose, lactic acid (E270), lactic acid esters (E472b), calcium lactate (E327), milk solids, skimmed milk powder, sodium lactate (E325), whey or whey solids.

If you are tempted to try alternative dairy sources, such as goat's or ewe's milk, bear in mind that biochemical analysis shows little difference between them and cow's milk, except in the level of protein. Nevertheless, some sufferers do report a difference when switching to another type of milk, so this is an option worth considering.

Before ruling out dairy foods completely, remember that milk, butter, cream and many cheeses can be high in fat. And high fat alone will trigger symptoms in some people (see below). So if you react to dairy products it might be the fat content, rather than the lactose, that is triggering or exacerbating your symptoms. If you think you are sensitive to milk, see how you react to skimmed milk, which has most of the ingredients of full-fat milk (including lactose) but not the fat, before giving them up completely.

Fat and IBS

The presence of food in the stomach triggers a wave of contraction called a mass movement, which pushes waste matter through the bowel. This is the gastrocolic reflex and is strongest in the morning. This is why many people get the urge to go to the toilet around 30–40 minutes after breakfast. High-fat foods provoke a stronger reaction in the digestive tract than low- or non-fat foods. This is because the strength of the signal produced by chemoreceptors in the gut (and the bowel's response to them) is related, in part, to the calories in a meal. Fat has double the calories of protein or carbohydrate and so causes a much stronger reaction, such as more powerful muscular contractions.

For IBS sufferers, a fatty meal causes such an extreme reaction that contractions become abnormal, leading to abdominal pain and constipation/diarrhoea. It may seem bizarre that this causes diarrhoea and constipation, but the bowel's squeezing and pushing movements (peristalsis) work correctly only when intestinal muscles receive nerve signals in the right order and of the correct intensity. Irregular signals upset the rhythm, causing excessive bowel movements and diarrhoea, or sluggish motions and constipation.

In a study reported to the American College of Gastroenterology, a strong connection was made between IBS and a high-fat diet. The study, carried out at the Mayo Clinic in Scotsdale, Arizona, involved 221 patients aged from 20 to 50, over 90 per cent of whom had IBS, functional dyspepsia or both. The patients were found to consume a significantly higher amount of fat, but less carbohydrate, than non-sufferers.

This would suggest that a change to a lower-fat higher-carbohydrate diet can be helpful in the management of IBS (as well as making good health sense in general). The message to the conference was that IBS sufferers should avoid making blanket changes in their diet, but should try to identify problem foods and limit their intake – or cut them out altogether – taking care not to rule out important food groups in the process.

Food Sensitivity

Most sufferers report that symptoms can be triggered or made worse by certain foods. Apart from wheat and dairy foods, the ones most likely to cause problems include caffeine (especially in coffee), fructose (fruit sugar, especially in dried fruit and fruit juice), citrus fruits, cabbages and pulses. Around 20 per cent of sufferers have noticed symptoms after eating potatoes.

Caffeine
In some IBS sufferers, caffeine causes diarrhoea, spasms and abdominal pain, and an urgent desire to go to the lavatory. Even decaffeinated coffee can cause this, but whether as a direct chemical effect or a psychological association with coffee drinking is unclear. This mildly addictive chemical is also found in tea, chocolate and some fizzy drinks, such as colas, and is added to cakes desserts and many painkillers. You will need to study the labels on all the products you buy in order to avoid this ubiquitous substance. However, simply reducing your intake by, for example, limiting the number of cups of coffee you drink may reduce the frequency and severity of symptoms without your needing to avoid caffeine altogether.

Cabbage Family
Some IBS sufferers find that symptoms such as bloating, excess wind and abdominal pain are worse after eating cruciferous vegetables: for example, cabbage, broccoli, cauliflower and Brussel sprouts. The cabbage family can generate excess wind in most people, including non-IBS sufferers. But symptoms are often more extreme in those with IBS.

Many sufferers choose to avoid cruciferous vegetables completely. But that means missing out on their many health-giving qualities. They are rich in vitamins C, E and folate, and minerals such as calcium, iron and potassium. They also contain sulphur compounds with important anti-cancer properties. A better approach is to reduce your intake to the point where symptoms are tolerable. Around 30 g (1 oz) of cruciferous vegetables per day, on average, provide optimum benefits without causing problems.

Problems with Pulses
Similarly, beans and other pulses, such as peas, lentils and chickpeas, cause excess gas and bloating in some sufferers. However, pulses are an excellent source of protein. Vegetarians, in particular, should include pulses in the diet in order to get the full range of amino acids (the building blocks of protein) the body needs for health. If you find that beans are a problem food, persevere but try reducing your intake until symptoms ease.

Other Problem Foods
Red and green peppers, which contain the spice capsaicin, and foods such as curries and pizzas that often include these vegetables, can also be problematic for IBS sufferers. Dried fruits, such as raisins and sultanas, may have been treated with sulphur dioxide (E220), known to cause IBS symptoms. (Sulphur dioxide is also found in wine.)

Citrus fruits – oranges, lemons, limes, satsumas, mandarins and clementines, and the drinks and desserts made from them – are another potential problem food. In part, this may be because of their high acid content, which may trigger the hypersensitive receptors in the gut. These foods are also high in sugar, which encourages excess growth of the yeast fungus candida, and so may also cause candidiasis (see Chapter Four). If candida infection may be a factor in your symptoms, try to limit sugary foods, at least temporarily, until candida is under control.

IBS and Amines
A group of chemicals called 'amines' is currently being studied as a potential cause of IBS symptoms. A subgroup, the biogenic amines, occur naturally in food or are made by the body from certain food ingredients. These include histamine, phenylethylamine, serotonin, tryptophan and tyramine. Some biogenic amines, most notably serotonin and histamine, act as signalling molecules in the body. Histamine, in particular, triggers many of the symptoms we associate with allergies. Biogenic amines are associated with many of the foods found to trigger IBS symptoms in some people, including cheese, chocolate, citrus fruit, eggs, shellfish, tomatoes and wine.

Another group, the heterocyclic amines (HCAs), are produced when foods are cooked at high temperatures. Toasted bread, meat-based gravy and grilled, fried or barbecued meat all contain high levels of HCAs. In some people, IBS symptoms arising from eating toast or beef, for example, may be interpreted as intolerance to those foods when the cause could be a sensitivity to the HCAs formed by the cooking process. Steaming and microwaving food is not thought to produce significant levels of HCAs.

Keeping a Food Diary

In order to manage IBS effectively, it is important to identify which foods may be triggering symptoms. You can then cut down on these foods to the point where they no longer cause problems, or, if necessary, eliminate them altogether. The list of foods that may trigger IBS symptoms is seemingly endless, so you will need to take a systematic approach. One method is to keep a food diary. A desk diary or large notebook will do, and make each page a separate day. Divide each page into columns. In the first column write down everything you have eaten and drunk that day and at what time of day.

Include snacks and other refreshments consumed between meals, such as biscuits, sweets, crisps, cakes, tea, coffee and colas, and not just main meals. Medicines, such as painkillers, can also be culprits, so make a note of them, too.

In the next column, write down any symptoms that you may attribute to IBS. In addition to the most common symptoms, such as diarrhoea/constipation, abdominal pain, bloating and flatulence, this column might also include less common problems that you hadn't previously associated with your IBS, such as an unpleasant feeling of fullness after meals, passing water frequently, headaches/migraine and depression.

It is also important to have a separate column to record psychological/emotional factors that might be contributing to your symptoms. Likely candidates include heavy workload, tight deadlines, impending exams, weddings and other stressful events, rows and other conflicts with work colleagues or managers, and illness or relationship problems involving friends, partners, family members or other relatives. This helps ensure that harmless foods are not wrongly blamed for symptoms triggered by your emotional state. It also helps to identify stress factors that exacerbate symptoms and should encourage you to take steps to deal with them (see Chapter Eleven).

Identifying Problem Foods

Once you have kept a food diary for a few weeks you should be able to identify foods most closely linked to symptoms. Bear in mind, though, that some potential problem foods often appear in combination. For example, a cup of coffee might also contain milk, and if you like your beverages sweet, sugar as well. Each of these ingredients may cause symptoms. So if you think coffee might be a problem, for example, and you normally drink it with milk, try to confirm your suspicions by drinking it black for a while or try an alternative to dairy milk, such as soya or rice milk, to see if that makes a difference.

If you choose carefully you can avoid problem foods and wait to see if your symptoms improve. If this seems to solve your problems, and you are happy to omit these foods from your diet on a permanent basis, then that is probably your best option.

If you want to confirm that these foods cause symptoms, you could reintroduce them one at a time – leaving a gap of several days between each one – to see if your symptoms recur. If they do, this would seem to prove your suspicions were correct.

Elimination Diet

If you are finding it difficult identifying problem foods, or you want to take a more systematic approach, you can try an elimination diet. This means following a simple diet for two to three weeks while avoiding suspect foods to see if this makes a difference to your symptoms. A suitable bland diet could include white fish (unsmoked), fresh garden vegetables (steamed, microwaved or boiled), water and herbal drinks, such as chamomile, not thought to cause dietary problems in most people. This rules out the most common culprits, such as wheat, dairy foods, citrus fruits, caffeinated drinks and alcohol. If you see a reduction in your symptoms, reintroduce suspect foods one at a time (leaving a gap of several days between each one) to see whether symptoms return.

A diet like this can be difficult to persevere with. If you feel the urge to snack between meals, opt for healthy choices that are not likely to trigger symptoms. For example, pieces of fresh raw vegetable and rice crackers are less problematic. Avoid crisps and biscuits that are high in fat, sugar or salt, as these can cause problems.

You may identify a problem food you would prefer not to cut out of your diet completely. As with caffeine, cruciferous vegetables and pulses, IBS sufferers often find they can tolerate a limited amount of problem foods without suffering symptoms. This is a useful approach as it reduces the risk that you are eliminating vital food groups. It also means that you may not need to avoid tea, coffee, alcohol and other stimulants, just moderate your intake.

Where possible, try to replace problem foods with products that contain similar amounts of the same nutrients. For example, milk is a good source of calcium. If you need to avoid it, consider switching to soya milk, which is fortified with calcium and so makes a good substitute (bear in mind, though, that some people are sensitive/allergic to soya products).

Most health food shops also stock dietary enzymes such as lactase, amylase (to break down starch), lipase (for fats) and protease (for proteins) to aid digestion in those who think they may be lacking them.

Professional Advice

IBS sufferers are generally well fed, fit and healthy (apart from their IBS symptoms) and so are well placed to carry out an elimination diet. However, if you find you are eliminating too many foods or food groups from your diet, without finding suitable alternatives, you may be running the risk of nutritional deficiencies. In this case it is advisable to consult a registered dietician. Your doctor can recommend a suitable professional or refer you to one directly. The dietician can prepare a diet plan tailored to your needs, enabling you to avoid problem foods while still ensuring that you are getting sufficient energy and the vital nutrients necessary for your age and gender.

Anyone who is pregnant or has an ongoing medical condition, such as diabetes mellitus, which requires them to follow a strict dietary regimen, should never change their diet without first consulting a doctor, dietician or other health care professional who is closely involved with the management of their condition.

Chapter Three

Boosting Good Bacteria

We carry around with us an incredible 1 kg (2.2 lb) of bacteria inside the bowel all the time – equivalent in weight to a bag of sugar. Over a year, we produce our own body weight in microbes. Most of these bacteria are harmless. Some are extremely beneficial but a minority, pathogens, cause disease. Common pathogens include strains of the bacteria *Clostridium, Campylobacter* and *Esherichia coli*, and the fungal yeast *Candida albicans*.

Studies carried out on healthy human volunteers show that our complement of bowel bacteria – good and bad – is highly individual, comprising about one hundred species. Maintaining the right balance between good and bad bacteria is crucial. Anything that disrupts the gut ecology (a condition called 'dysbiosis') can cause bowel symptoms, for pathogens multiply to harmful levels if not held in check by the beneficial types.

Friends from Birth

An unborn baby's bowel is completely sterile. The bacteria that take up residence there are derived from the mother during childbirth and then from the diet early in life. By two years old, colonization of the bowel is complete. After that, any alteration in bowel microflora arises through dietary changes, or factors such as illness or medication.

Breastfed babies have a healthier gut microflora than bottle-fed infants. In part, this may be because of the greater risk of contamination when preparing a feed (whereas breast milk is pure). But the main reason is that human breast milk contains important substances that promote the growth of beneficial bacteria (see 'Introducing Prebiotics', this chapter). As a result, breastfed babies are less prone to gastrointestinal upsets. Some formula-feed manufacturers now produce milk containing the bacteria-boosting components found in breast milk.

IBS and Bacteria

There is growing evidence that an imbalance in bowel microflora is a key factor in IBS (and other digestive disorders such as inflammatory bowel diseases). Many IBS symptoms may be directly attributable to pathogens. Some bacteria release toxins that irritate and 'sensitize' the bowel, triggering pain, diarrhoea and/or constipation.

Another factor may be that pathogens interfere with the way gas is neutralized in the bowel. Gas is a common waste product of all gut microbes, but some bacteria are able to convert this gas into more condensed forms, such as methane and hydrogen sulphide, or other substances such as acetate, that take up less room.

Based on the average person's daily food consumption, bowel bacteria should produce 25–30 litres of gas each day. Thanks to the sulphate-producers, acetogens and other types of bacteria, this huge volume of gas is reduced to a more manageable 5 litres. However, if the finely balanced microfloral ecology is disrupted, the amount of gas produced increases, leading to bloating and flatulence symptomatic of IBS.

Upsetting the Balance

Both 'good' and 'bad' bacteria are drastically reduced by antibiotics, but many pathogens are resistant to these drugs and so recover more quickly than beneficial types. In the United Kingdom, around one million people take antibiotic medication every week. This is 12 per cent of all prescription medications given to adults. In children, the figure is 27 per cent.

Older people have a greater problem. Past the age of 50, levels of friendly bacteria drop dramatically, just at a time when the protection they offer is needed most. This problem is particularly acute in elderly patients receiving antibiotic treatment. In hospitals and nursing homes, colonic infection with the pathogen *Clostridium difficile* following antibiotic treatment is a common cause of diarrhoea.

Whatever the reason for the decline in beneficial microbes, this allows pathogens to gain the upper hand. Autism is just one consequence of this. There is strong evidence that autism is due, at least in some cases, to neuro-toxins (brain poisons) produced by a strain of *Clostridium*. Many previously normal children first start to show signs of autism following antibiotic treatment. An obvious implication is that antibiotics neutralize beneficial bacteria, allowing *Clostridium* to multiply.

IBS and Infection

Clostridium and *Campylobacter* have both been implicated in IBS, and in other diseases such as ulcerative colitis, Crohn's disease and bowel cancer. For some IBS sufferers, symptoms may be triggered, or made worse, by *Candida albicans*. As with harmful bacteria, candida is normally kept down by good bacteria. You can do a lot to improve your IBS symptoms (and avoid the problem in the first place) by maintaining a healthy bowel environment. This includes reducing the risk of food poisoning and other gut infections (see Chapter Ten) and boosting levels of beneficial bacteria.

Friendly Bacteria – What Do They Do?

Beneficial bacteria have many important roles. As well as reducing the amount of gas in the gut they also help metabolize (break down) food efficiently, reducing the risk of food allergies and intolerances (see Chapter Two). Friendly bacteria also produce important organic acids, such as acetate, and butyric and propionic acids. Acetate is turned into the energy compound ATP. Up to 10 per cent of a healthy person's energy needs may be met by bacteria in this way. Butyric acid fuels cells of the bowel (colonocytes) and helps prevent bowel cancer. Propionic acid reduces cholesterol production in the liver, so guarding against heart disease. Bacteria even produce vital nutrients like vitamin B2 and K.

Protecting us against pathogens is probably their most important function. They:

- form colonies that expand and crowd out pathogens (colonization resistance).
- prevent pathogens attaching to the gut wall.
- compete for nutrients so there is less for pathogens.
- produce acids including hydrogen peroxide that lower the pH (raise the acidity) of the bowel to a level pathogens cannot tolerate.
- produce chemicals (bacteriocins) that destroy pathogens and the toxins they produce (including those that cause cancer).
- stimulate antibodies (immunoglobulins) and T-cells of the immune system to fight pathogens.

Introducing Probiotics

You can boost the beneficial bacteria in your gut by consuming 'probiotic' products. The two most important groups of friendly bacteria are bifidobacteria and *Lactobacillus*. Both can be found in many of the probiotic yoghurts and yoghurt drinks sold in large stores, and as tablets, capsules and powders available from good health food shops, by mail order or on the Internet.

The term 'probiotic' was coined by Professor Glenn Gibson of Reading University. He has spent many years researching gut ecology and has carried out studies supporting a link between bacteria and health. Using an arrangement of glass containers and tubes nicknamed 'roboguts', Professor Gibson has duplicated healthy and unhealthy digestive systems, from infancy to old age, to study the effect of probiotics on bowel disorders.

The title of 'father of probiotics', even if he didn't use the word himself, should go to Nobel Prize winner Elie Metchnikoff, a Russian scientist working early last century. Metchnikoff studied Bulgarian mountain peasants and attributed their longevity and health to a tradition of eating fermented milk products on a daily basis. Metchnikoff published a report of his findings in 1908 stating his belief that yoghurt bacteria support a healthy gut microflora, and that this improves health and wellbeing.

The current interest in probiotic drinks can be attributed to a Japanese doctor, Minoru Shirota, founder of the Yakult company. In 1938, he isolated the strain of gut bacteria named after him – *Lactobacillus casei* Shirota. This was added to a milk drink and initially given to patients at his health clinic. Japan is the world's top consumer of probiotics.

What to Look For

Most traditional yoghurts contain two principal species of lactic acid bacteria: *Lactobacillus delbrueckii* subsp. *bulgaricus* and *Streptococcus thermophilus*. These are called 'starter cultures' because they instigate the fermentation process that gives yoghurt its distinctive taste and texture. However, traditional strains of yoghurt bacteria are not particularly resistant to gastric acids, and it is unclear how many survive the journey through the digestive tract long enough to reach and colonize the gut.

To get to the bowel, probiotics must pass through many barriers, not only stomach acids, but also bile salts and other pancreatic secretions. Many friendly bacteria are destroyed along the way. Probiotic cultures in yoghurts, drinks and supplements often contain tougher species, either occurring naturally in the bowel or specially bred to survive the adverse conditions of the GI tract and take up residence in the bowel. They include:

- *Bifidobacterium breve*
- *Bifidobacterium bifidum*
- *Bifidobacterium essensis*
- *Bifidobacterium digestivum*
- *Bifidobacterium lactis*
- *Bifidobacterium longum*
- *Lactobacillus acidophilus*
- *Lactobacillus casei*
- *Lactobacillus plantarum*
- *Lactobacillus rhamnosus GG*
- *Lactobacillus reuteri*
- *Lactobacillus tacidophilus*
- *Saccharomyces boulardii* (a probiotic yeast)

More probiotic microbes are appearing all the time. Of these, *Lactobacillus plantarum* is thought to be particularly effective against candida infection. If you are taking antibiotics, it is important to take probiotics, especially capsules, as soon as the course is finished to repopulate the bowel before the pathogens gain a foothold. You can now obtain supplements containing *Bifidobacterium infanta*, the strain of bacterium found in breastfed infants but often lacking in bottle-fed babies. It helps guard against digestive ailments common in non-breastfed infants – and may help prevent autism.

Choosing Probiotics

Many modern yoghurts and yoghurt drinks are made in the traditional way and pasteurized to kill off the original bacteria. Hardy strains of probiotic bacteria are then added. When buying probiotic foods, check that the product states 'live bacteria' or 'probiotic' somewhere on the packaging.

Some brands are sold heat-treated (marked 'pasteurized', 'sterilized', 'long-life' or 'UHT') without the later addition of live cultures. Heat treatment kills the cultures so these foods have only limited probiotic effect, but may still be of value (see below).

Several studies, including one published in 2004 and conducted by Professor Jeremy Hamilton-Miller of the Department of Medical Microbiology, Royal Free Hospital, London, cast doubt on some probiotic products. Professor Hamilton-Miller and his team formulated the following criteria for probiotic products. They must:

- include strains of beneficial microbes hardy enough to survive gastric acids and other digestive juices and pass through to the bowel where they can become established.
- comprise strains of beneficial microbes that attach firmly enough to the bowel wall to avoid being carried out of the GI tract by the daily passage of gut contents.
- contain beneficial microbes in sufficient numbers to form viable colonies.
- be stable enough to allow the microbes to survive during the shelf life of the product and to continue to be effective right up to the expiry date.
- have clear, accurate and informative labelling regarding the contents of the product.

Professor Hamilton-Miller's team studied 52 probiotic brands in three categories – supplements, fermented functional foods, and health care products. In some cases, the labelling was inaccurate and health claims unproven. A few products did not contain the probiotic bacteria listed, and – of more concern – contained unlisted bacteria (such as *Enterococcus faecium*, a potential pathogen). But most products satisfied some or all of the team's requirements.

The researchers only studied microbes in laboratory conditions. No attempt was made to study their effectiveness in humans or other living creatures. Also the criteria that Professor Hamilton-Miller's team laid down were their own. One Finnish study, however, suggests that yoghurt need not necessarily contain live bacteria in order to have beneficial effects. A group from the University of Turku, in Finland, led by Tanja Pessi discovered that probiotic bacteria contain substances that stimulate the immune system whether alive, dead or fragmented.

By consuming a range of good-quality probiotic products you can increase the likelihood of success. Yoghurts and yoghurt drinks contain many important nutrients apart from their bacterial content, such as calcium and lactic acid. A good way to take probiotics is in 'enteric coated' capsules, which are resistant to stomach acids and release the good bacteria only in the bowel, where they take up residence.

Including Probiotics in the Diet

Many probiotic yoghurts are sweetened. Unsweetened types have a sharp, acidic taste produced by natural fermentation and may not be to everyone's liking. These can be made more palatable by serving with fruit and desserts. Plain probiotic yoghurts can also be mixed into smoothies, stirred into soups and stews (allow to cool first) or flavoured with herbs, spices and seasonings such as mustard or garlic and used as a salad dressing or a topping for jacket potatoes. Chapter Nine contains suggestions for introducing live yoghurt into your meals. All probiotic products should be served unheated as oven cooking or microwaving kills the beneficial bacteria they contain.

Some IBS sufferers with a sensitivity/intolerance to dairy products may not be able to consume probiotic yoghurt, perhaps because of a deficiency of the lactase needed to digest lactose in dairy foods (see Chapter Two). In this case, soya-based yoghurts, or tablets, powders and other non-yoghurt sources of probiotics, might be more suitable.

Although dairy products in general can cause digestive upsets, live yoghurt is usually well tolerated in all but the most sensitive people. There may be two principal reasons for this. First, micro-organisms in yoghurt also produce lactase. Second, yoghurt is thicker and more viscous than milk and so stays in the gut longer, allowing more time for lactose digestion.

Introducing 'Prebiotics

Friendly bacteria introduced via the diet may diminish in the gut over time unless topped up with regular consumption of probiotic products. Another approach, combined with (not instead of) probiotics is to encourage these bacteria by feeding them the special nutrients they need. This method is called 'prebiotics', again a term coined by Professor Gibson. Bifidobacteria and *Lactobacillus* thrive on a type of fibre made up of short chains of sugar molecules called 'oligosaccharides' ('oligo' means 'few' and 'saccharide' means 'sugar'). It tastes sweet but is different from sucrose (table sugar).

The human digestive system does not produce the enzymes needed to digest this fibre, so it passes through to the bowel largely unchanged. Once there it nourishes the good bacteria, enabling them to multiply, but without boosting the pathogens which lack the enzymes needed to break it down. There are several types of oligosaccharides: fructo-oligosaccharides (better known as FOS), galacto-oligosaccharides (GOS), inulin and lactulose.

FOS consists of short chains of fructose (fruit sugar) molecules, strung together. FOS and inulin are the most common oligosaccharides found naturally in foods. Chicory contains exceptionally high levels. FOS is also found in the following fruits, vegetables and cereals:

- artichoke
- asparagus
- banana
- barley
- burdock
- corn
- garlic
- leeks
- oats
- olives
- onion
- peas
- wholewheat

Galacto-oligosaccharides are short chains of galactose molecules, derived from lactose, present in milk (especially human breast milk, thus promoting beneficial bacteria in infants) and dairy foods such as yoghurt. GOS is also found in soya products, such as soya milk, tofu and tempeh. Soya milk makes a good substitute for dairy milk for those with lactose sensitivity/intolerance. Lactulose is another prebiotic oligosaccharide. It acts as a laxative when taken in large quantities but at lower doses can promote probiotic bacteria.

How Much Prebiotic Do I Need?
The average person gets about 2 g of FOS from a balanced, healthy diet with lots of fruit and vegetables. For maximum benefit, intake should increase to

at least 5 g. This is difficult to achieve through food alone. But you can also get FOS supplements as capsules, tablets and powders, often mixed with probiotic bacteria. These are available from health food shops, mail order companies and Internet sites. Food manufacturers are also introducing prebiotics to staple foods including bread, breakfast cereals, margarine, drinks and salad dressing.

FOS Powder
FOS is a versatile product, especially as a powder. It is about half as sweet as table sugar but without the calories. Nor does it encourage candidiasis (see Chapter Four) or other fungal infections. FOS can be sprinkled on cereal, desserts such as fresh fruit or crumbles, or blended into yoghurt or fruit juice. See Chapter Nine for more delicious ways to use FOS. As a soluble fibre, it also promotes healthy bowel function.

It may not be suitable for those taking any medication that would be inhibited by agents that lower the pH (increase acidity levels) in the gut. If you are receiving medication, seek a doctor's or pharmacist's advice before using FOS. It is also quite expensive. Hopefully, the price will fall as it becomes more widely used.

Biotic Bonus
Unlike many medications for IBS, few side effects have been reported with prebiotic and probiotic foods and supplements. In some people, flatulence may increase for a while, although this will diminish over time. High intakes of FOS (40 g and over) may cause diarrhoea. People with compromised immune systems should seek medical advice before taking probiotics, because of the potential (although slight) risk of infection. The most serious side effect of prebiotics reported is an allergy to inulin experienced by a 39-year-old man who had consumed large doses of supplements, obtained from several sources. This condition is extremely rare.

Preventing Disease
This preventive approach is so effective that pre- and probiotic foods have been introduced at children's day care facilities, and old people's homes, to help prevent the spread of common infections, including rotavirus. Regular use of pre- and probiotics also aids absorption of calcium and magnesium, which helps guard against the brittle bone condition osteoporosis. Other studies indicate that probiotic supplementation helps control blood sugar levels in diabetics, and reduces abnormally high blood-fat levels.

Future Probiotic Foods

Although prebiotic and probiotic products are well established in Japan and in parts of Europe, in the United Kingdom and the United States, manufacturers are only now recognizing the potential market for functional foods. At the time of writing the range of products most widely available was mainly limited to various types of fermented foods, but new brands can be expected over the coming months and years.

One product with potential as a probiotic functional food is cheese. It is effective at supporting probiotic bacteria and delivering them safely to the gut without adverse effects on the flavour or texture of the cheese. Currently under development are prebiotic/probiotic milks, frozen yoghurt and ice cream, but many other foods could also be adapted to incorporate a 'functional' element.

Medicinal Probiotics

The medicinal use of probiotic tablets, capsules and powders (called 'biotherapy') is likely to increase significantly. In one study of elderly hospital patients, subjects receiving probiotic therapy comprising capsules of *Lactobacillus acidophilus* and *Bifidobacterium bifidum* had much lower rates of *Clostridium difficile* infection than those taking dummy (placebo) capsules. Some strains of probiotic bacteria, such as *Lactobacillus rhamnosus GG*, *Bifidobacterium longum* and the probiotic yeast *Saccharomyces boulardii* help prevent antibiotic-related diarrhoea and reduce the incidence of rotavirus, a leading cause of gastroenteritis in infants worldwide.

Doctors may use probiotics for food allergies and conditions such as high blood pressure and high cholesterol levels, in the treatment of bladder infections and in cancer prevention. Because of their ability to stimulate the immune system and aid disease resistance, probiotics may reduce the need for antibiotics.

Chapter Four

Candida and Sugar

When tested, many IBS sufferers were found to have the pathogenic yeast *Candida albicans* in the digestive tract, crucially, at levels above that found in non-sufferers. Whether this shows that candida is a major contributory factor in IBS, or an opportunist taking advantage of the microfloral imbalance to multiply and spread, is unclear.

Candida is responsible for the troublesome condition candidiasis (better known as thrush), which affects the digestive tract, vagina and, less often, mouth and throat, especially in infants, the elderly and those with a badly compromised immune system. Other, much less common, variations include candidiasis of the skin and nails. Even more rarely, the disease may spread throughout the body, causing a potentially fatal condition called 'systemic thrush'.

What Causes Candida Infection?

Candida is normally present in relatively low numbers on the mucous membranes that line the mouth, vagina and bowel. Most of the time candida does little harm because it is kept in check by the beneficial bacteria also present. However, any change in conditions that tips the balance in favour of the yeast can lead to a sudden rapid rise in candida numbers. It is this increase, or 'overgrowth', in yeast cells that causes symptoms.

Common factors thought to contribute to yeast infection include:

- decline in the friendly bacteria that normally suppress candida, for example, following a course of antibiotics or corticosteroid drugs.
- change in pH (acid/alkaline) balance of the mucous membranes, for example, through a change in diet. A high-sugar diet causes pH to rise, leading to more alkaline conditions, which suits candida. Bacteria prefer a slightly acid environment, so their numbers are suppressed.
- illness, resulting in lowered resistance to infection, which allows candida to multiply.

Diabetes mellitus increases the risk of contracting all forms of candida infection. Even when diabetes is well-controlled, blood sugar (glucose) levels are consistently higher than in non-diabetics. Pregnancy and the use of oral contraceptives cause changes in hormonal levels that can also raise blood sugar levels and so raise pH.

How Candida Spreads

Candida normally exists as a relatively benign round yeast form, but under certain circumstances it converts to pathogenic finger-like rhizoids, which infiltrate and inflame the bowel wall, disrupting the normal functioning of the digestive tract.

The rhizoids feed on carbohydrates, especially sugars, and convert them into different substances, including acetaldehyde (a nerve toxin), carbon dioxide (a common waste gas) and even alcohol. These substances not only act on the bowel, but also spread via the bloodstream to the liver, kidneys and brain, where they can have other potentially serious effects. For example, they can interfere with the liver's ability to eliminate toxins from the body. Candida infection also suppresses the immune system, allowing parasitic organisms such as *Giardia lamblia*, *Entamoeba histolytica* and *Blastocystic hominis* to gain a foothold, further aggravating digestive symptoms.

Candida and IBS

A direct link between candida infection and IBS symptoms is unproven, but it is likely that candida overgrowth is common in IBS sufferers who have had antibiotic treatment. Many antibiotics have a 'broad spectrum' effect. This means they destroy both disease organisms and harmless microbes – including beneficial bacteria.

Candida, like all fungi, is generally unaffected by antibiotics, so the sudden rapid decline in 'friendly' bacteria leaves the way clear for candida to multiply and colonize large areas of the gut. The presence of candida, and the toxins it produces, may be enough to sensitize the gut lining and trigger, or exacerbate, symptoms.

In time, the beneficial bacteria increase in numbers and re-establish themselves, and so regain control over candida. However, any factor that favours candida and not the beneficial bacteria, such as a high-sugar diet, allows the yeast to proliferate in the gut.

How Can I Tackle Candida?

If there is a link between candidiasis and IBS (and even if unproven, it seems a plausible scenario), it follows that managing the condition may help tackle symptoms. This is best approached in two ways. The first, as explained in Chapter Three, is to promote the development of beneficial bacteria, for example by regularly consuming probiotic drinks, yoghurt and supplements, and by eating prebiotic foods and supplements such as FOS that support a healthy gut flora. The second is to follow a low-sugar diet that discourages candida overgrowth. This two-pronged attack should restore the balance in the gut, allowing beneficial bacteria to regain control.

Sugar and Processed Foods
Along with salt, sugar is the most common food additive in the Western diet. Most sugar is derived from two main sources – sugar cane and sugar beet. These are crushed to release sugar syrup, which is then boiled and processed to produce familiar forms such as molasses (treacle), granulated, caster and icing and brown sugar.

Molasses is unrefined sugar, and is a source of magnesium (2.5 mg per 1 g). To make white granulated sugar, this raw product is passed through a charcoal filter, dried and then ground into granules. Caster sugar is granulated sugar ground fine, and icing is ground even finer. Brown sugar is white sugar with a little molasses added for colour.

Increasingly, manufacturers are looking to alternative sources to provide the sugar used in processed foods. For example, fructose, in its natural form, is found in fruit and vegetables (although it can be processed from cane and beet sugar). It is also found in large quantities in fruit juice (especially concentrates) and dried fruit. Corn syrup (a type of fructose) is derived from cornstarch, dextrose (a type of glucose) comes from corn syrup, and grape sugar (a type of fructose) comes – unsurprisingly – from grapes.

Sugar is added to a wide range of processed products, usually in the form of sucrose, dextrose and fructose. Fructose is particularly sweet, hence its inclusion in so many processed foods. High levels of sugar are found not only in sweet items, such as biscuits, cakes, desserts, and tinned and frozen fruit, as you might expect, but also in savoury foods such as burger buns, baked beans, ketchup, and pasta and chilli sauces.

Sugar and Health
A good case can be made for limiting consumption of sugary foods, for reasons quite apart from managing candida. Sugar added to food represents 'empty' calories. It supplies energy, and so contributes to the problem of excess weight, but without the vitamins, minerals (with the exception of magnesium in molasses), fibre and other important nutrients found naturally in fruit and vegetables.

Eating high-sugar foods can lead to abnormal fluctuations in blood sugar levels. This can cause a sugar 'rush', a hyperactive state rapidly followed by sudden fatigue. High sugar consumption is one factor blamed for a rise in type II diabetes, a condition once seen mainly in older people but now increasingly common in the young.

Even natural, unsweetened juices are problematic. When consumed on an empty stomach their high sugar content passes rapidly through the gut wall and into the bloodstream, again causing a rapid rise in blood sugar.

Sugar inhibits the ability of leukocytes (white blood cells) and other components of the immune system to counteract bacterial infection. Several studies involving healthy volunteers have shown that the antibacterial action of immune cells is reduced for several hours following a high sucrose meal. This may be another factor contributing to an imbalance in the gut flora, enabling candida and other pathogenic microbes to thrive.

Fructose and IBS

There is growing evidence of an association between IBS and fructose. One study, carried out at the University of Iowa, involved a group of 80 patients with suspected IBS who were tested for fructose intolerance (difficulty digesting this sugar). Of these, 30 tested 'positive'. This group was put on a diet that restricted their consumption of fruit and fructose-rich foods and, according to the investigators, noticed a significant reduction in symptoms such as abdominal pain, bloating and diarrhoea.

In a follow-up study, those patients interviewed who had remained on a fructose-restricted diet continued to report a reduction in symptoms, while those who reverted to their normal diet reported no improvement in their condition. The same researchers had previously carried out studies which, they said, indicated that up to 60 per cent of IBS sufferers may have fructose intolerance. Some doctors question whether patients in the study really had IBS to start with. Others doubt the existence of 'fructose intolerance'.

Another problem sugar, sorbitol, found, for example, in diet products, has also been implicated in IBS. But as with fructose, the exact link remains unclear.

Controlling Sugar Intake

It is possible to limit your sugar intake simply by avoiding processed foods, especially soft drinks, cakes, biscuits and puddings that contain high levels of sugar. You should also avoid adding sugar to tea and coffee, and try limiting the amount you add to your cooking. The sugar content of processed foods, usually listed as sucrose, dextrose, fructose, glucose, corn syrup or invert sugar (a form of sucrose processed to make it sweeter), is listed on the packaging.

In the short term, say two or three weeks, you could try avoiding all sugary foods, including citrus fruits, dried fruits and other high-sugar fruits – and the juices made from them. In the longer term, there is no need to miss out on the health benefits that fruit and fruit juices can provide. But it is a good idea to enjoy them with a balanced meal. The fibre, fat and protein in the meal will slow the passage of sugar into the bloodstream, and so help normalize blood sugar levels. Avoid having sugary drinks on their own too often, as they not only pass into the bloodstream too rapidly, but also into the bowel.

Fresh fruits are important components of a healthy, balanced diet, containing soluble and in some cases insoluble fibre, as well as the all-important vitamins, minerals and phyto-chemicals. So even if you decide to cut out fruit for a while to limit your intake of fructose, it is a good idea to reintroduce it into your diet as soon as you start to notice an improvement in symptoms.

Other Dietary Changes
In addition to cutting back on sugary foods, nutritionists suggest avoiding all refined carbohydrates, including white bread and other processed-flour products, such as biscuits, pastries and cakes, white rice and processed pasta. Instead, include more wholegrain foods such as wholemeal bread, wholemeal pasta and brown rice.

Some nutritionists also suggest reducing your intake of foods produced by fermentation, such as bread, blue-veined cheeses, yeast-based spreads, stock cubes and soy sauce, smoked or salty foods, such as smoked meats and fish, caffeinated drinks, such as tea, coffee and colas, and alcohol.

In place of these foods, you could try a diet that includes plenty of raw and lightly cooked vegetables, brown rice, fish, live yoghurt, garlic, olive oil and herbal teas. Whether or not a diet like this can control candida overgrowth in the gut, it has much to commend it on general health grounds (in the short term only).

Beneficial Biotin
Biotin, one of the B complex of vitamins, may play a role in the natural control of candida. This vitamin is produced by some forms of gut bacteria, as well as being a component of many foods. In the healthy gut, biotin may help prevent candida switching from its harmless yeast form to the aggressive rhizoid sub-type. To benefit from this protective effect, include more natural sources of biotin in the diet, such as

wholegrains, peas, beans (including soya), fruit, nuts, eggs, mushrooms and cauliflower.

Oestrogen can inhibit absorption of biotin, so women taking oestrogen-based contraceptive pills or hormonal replacement therapy (HRT) might gain particular benefit by increasing their intake of biotin-rich foods and/or taking biotin supplements.

Chapter Five

IBS and Additives

There are over four hundred additives approved for food use, with more under consideration. In Europe most additives are given an international E number so they can be identified in each member country, regardless of the national language and the name by which that additive is known locally.

Additives range from complex compounds such as polyoxyethylene sorbitan monooleate (E433) to simple elements such as oxygen (E948) and hydrogen (E949). Some additives are also found naturally in foods, such as vitamin C (ascorbic acid, E300) and vitamin B3 (nicotinic acid/ nicotinamide, E375). Even precious metals – silver (E174) and gold (E175) – can be added to food and so require their own E number.

The role of additives

Food producers and manufacturers include additives for many reasons. For example, additives:

- enhance the look of food (colourings)
- enhance the taste of food (flavourings and flavour enhancers)
- help oily and watery foods to mix (emulsifiers)
- stop lumps forming in powdery foods (anti-caking agents)
- extend shelf-life by preventing food from going rancid (antioxidants)
- inhibit bacterial and fungal contamination (preservatives)
- pressurize food to force it out at the press of a button (gases/ propellants).

Many additives have more than one function. For example, nitrates act as both a preservative and a colouring. The majority of additives are regarded as safe for most people, and are not generally associated with symptoms. It is difficult to avoid them completely, and in any case most people prefer not to shun all additive-containing foods. But some additives are more problematic than others. They include chemicals known (or strongly suspected) to cause symptoms such as headaches, migraines, tight chest, nausea and allergic rashes, and conditions such as hyperactivity in children, and even blindness and neurodegenerative diseases such as

Alzheimer's and Parkinson's. Unfortunately, additives commonly associated with these problems include some of the most widely used colourings and flavour enhancers found in food today.

IBS and Additives

The connection between IBS and additives is unclear. Simply because an additive seems to trigger an unpleasant response, it does not mean that you are allergic to it. Nor does it follow that because an additive is thought to provoke a reaction in sensitive people it will trigger digestive symptoms in IBS sufferers.

But people with IBS are hypersensitive to all stimuli originating in the gut, and some additives may trigger a more powerful reaction than others. So it seems sensible to treat with caution those additives widely believed to provoke adverse reactions.

Some sufferers identify the additives they associate with symptoms. Others have found it difficult to find a direct link between IBS symptoms and a particular food, such as wheat, dairy or citrus fruits, but notice that some processed foods consistently trigger symptoms. So the possibility that additives are a contributory factor is worth exploring.

If you find that a food is causing symptoms yet does not contain an ingredient such as wheat, dairy food or fructose that you have found to be problematic before, it is worth looking at the list of additives to see whether the source of the trouble could be there.

You could use your food diary (see Chapter Two) to make a note of any E numbers associated with your symptoms on a regular basis. Of course, it may only be coincidence if you suffer abdominal pain or other symptoms after consuming a food containing an additive, but the more often a problem occurs, the stronger the likelihood of a link becomes.

High-risk Additives

For IBS sufferers, and others prone to food allergies or other adverse reactions to food, problematic additives include the sweetener aspartame, the flavour enhancer monosodium glutamate (MSG), the acidity regulator nicotinic acid, the glazing agent L-cysteine, and various preservatives, such as benzoic acid and its derivatives, sulphur dioxide, and colourings, especially those derived from azo dyes and coal tar.

Widespread Use

It is difficult to avoid the following additives altogether unless you choose to follow a very simple diet using only pure, unprocessed foods and shun all processed, smoked and pickled items. This is because additives can be found in a wide range of processed foods including one or more of the following: barbecue sauce, beer (including alcohol-free types), liqueurs and other alcoholic drinks, biscuits, blancmange, breadcrumbs, cakes (including cake mix and cake toppings), cheeses, chewing gum, chocolate, cocktail/glacé cherries, coffee essence, cold remedies, coleslaw, confectionery, cordials, crisps and other savoury snacks, cured meats, custard (powder and tinned), dressed crab, fish fingers, fish paste, fizzy drinks, flavoured yoghurt, frozen and packet desserts, fruit pureé, frying oil, garlic sausage, gravy granules, ice cream, ice lollies, icing, jam, jelly, lemon curd, low-calorie foods and drinks, low-calorie margarine, marmalade, marzipan, mayonnaise, meat balls, mint sauce, mustard, paté, pickled cucumbers, pie fillings, pies, pineapple juice, prawns, salad cream, salami, sauces, sausages, crisps and other savoury snacks, Scotch eggs, seafood sauces, smoked fish (including mackerel and kippers), soups (tinned and packet), soy sauce, spice blends, sponge cakes, squash, stuffed olives, tinned fruit, tinned peas and trifle.

Problem Additives
The following are some of the most controversial additives, but bear in mind that any additive may cause an adverse reaction, either individually or in combination.

Aspartame (E951)
One of the most common additives today, aspartame is popular with manufacturers because it is 200 times sweeter than table sugar but has few calories. It can be used on its own in tablet and granulated form as a low-calorie alternative to sugar in tea and coffee, and is added to many processed foods, especially desserts, preserves and drinks marked 'sugar-free', 'low-calorie', 'diet', 'light' and 'lite'.

Once inside the body, aspartame is broken down into a number of different substances, some with known or potentially harmful effects such as phenylalanine, aspartic acid, methanol (alcohol) and formaldehyde (embalming fluid).

Phenylalanine poses a serious threat to children with the congenital metabolic disorder phenylketonuria (PKU). These children cannot metabolize phenylalanine and suffer serious brain damage. By law, all foods (but not medicines) that contain aspartame must carry a warning stating 'contains a source of phenylalanine'.

Aspartame is a proven excitotoxin. These are chemicals that cause nerve cells to fire in the absence of a normal stimulus. It not only sensitizes tastebuds, so heightening its effect on the palate, but also stimulates nerve cells elsewhere in the body, including the brain and the lining of the bowel. Aspartame can cause abdominal pain and headache, and may exert toxic effects on brain cells (especially in a foetus). At the time of writing it was being investigated as a potential cause of brain tumour.

Monosodium Glutamate (E621)
Most commonly associated with Chinese meals, monosodium glutamate (MSG) is one of the most common flavour enhancers used in savoury foods including crisps, packet soups, pies, cured meats, sausages and sauces. It is chemically related to another flavour enhancer, glutamic acid (E620), now withdrawn from use in baby foods because of concern over potential brain damage. Like aspartame, MSG is an excitotoxin, and so has an excitatory effect on nerve cells and nerve endings, including those in the gut wall.

Symptoms associated with MSG include abdominal pain and nausea, burning and tingling sensations, chest pain and pressure, heart palpitations, dizziness, migraine, nerve tingling, excessive thirst, panic attacks, sweating and mood swings. In some people, MSG causes an acute hypersensitivity reaction called Kwok's disease (or 'Chinese restaurant syndrome'), named after Dr Robert Ho Man Kwok, who identified the condition in 1968.

Depending on sensitivity, symptoms can occur immediately or up to two days after ingesting the substance. MSG is also being investigated for a possible link with the eye disorder glaucoma and blindness, and serious neurodegenerative diseases including Alzheimer's, Huntington's and Parkinson's.

Nicotinic Acid (E375)
Also known as vitamin B3, nicotinic acid is an important nutrient that plays a vital role in energy metabolism and in the healthy functioning of the nervous and digestive systems. It is found naturally in a wide range of foods including eggs, dairy products and meats such as liver, chicken and turkey. It is unlikely to cause problems if consumed from natural sources alone. However, it is also added to breakfast cereals, bread, flour and vitamin supplements, sometimes at levels much higher than would occur normally. As a food additive, it is associated with abdominal pain and headache and – at very high levels – eye disorders, gastric disorders and liver damage.

Benzoic Acid (E210)
Occurring naturally in many fruits and vegetables, benzoic acid has antibacterial and antifungal properties that make it a useful preservative in pickled and marinated foods, fruit juices, jam, spreads, salad dressings, sweet sauces, syrups, fizzy drinks and beer. In some people it may cause

abdominal pain, nausea and allergic reactions including nettle rash (urticaria). Asthmatics and others sensitive to aspirin may find that benzoic acid triggers or exacerbates their symptoms. Chemically related preservatives used in similar products include calcium benzoate (E213), potassium benzoate (E212) and sodium benzoate (E211).

Sulphur Dioxide (E220)
This is one of the most widespread preservatives found in foods and drinks. It may also appear on labels as sodium bisulphite, potassium bisulphite or just plain sulphite. Sulphur dioxide is found in beer, burgers, dried fruits (and cakes and other foods that contain them), fruit juices and concentrates, sauces and pickles, among other foods. It can trigger abdominal pain and diarrhoea, rashes and tight chest – especially in asthmatics and those sensitive to aspirin. Chemically related preservatives include sodium metabisulphite (E223), potassium metabisulphite (E224) and sodium benzoate (E211).

SunsetYellow (E110)
Along with tartrazine (E102), sunset yellow is arguably the most infamous of the azo dyes. These are red, brown and yellow pigments, derived from amino compounds, that turn foods and drinks a garish colour. For example, tartrazine makes food bright yellow. If mixed with synthetic coal tar dyes such as brilliant blue (E133) or green S (E142), foods turn bright green. Azo dyes are found in jelly, jam, ice cream, pie fillings, squash, sauces, soups and confectionery.

Azo dyes are associated with abdominal pain, nausea and other gastric upsets, and allergic reactions, such as nettle rash (urticaria), especially in those who are sensitive to aspirin. Other commonly used azo dyes that can provoke an adverse reaction in some people include yellow 2G (E107), carmoisine (E122), amaranth (E123), ponceau 4R (E124), red 2G (E128), allura red (E129), black PN (E151), brown FK (E154) and brown HT (E155).

Other azo dyes or synthetic coal tar dyes associated with abdominal disorders and/or allergies include quinoline yellow (E104), erythrosine (E127), patent blueV (E131), indigo carmine (E132), brilliant blue (E133) and green S (E142).

The following colourings (still common in the United Kingdom) are prohibited in the United States and parts of Europe: tartrazine, quinoline yellow, yellow 2G, carmoisine, amaranth, ponceau 4R, red 2G, brilliant blue FCF, green S, black PN, brown FK and brown HT.

Additives that may cause allergies

The following additives have been associated with allergies in some people.

Colourings

Allura Red AC	(E129)
Amaranth	(E123)
Azorubine / carmoisine	(E122)
Black 7984	(E152)
Brilliant Black BN, Black PN	(E151)
Brilliant Blue FCF	(E133)
Brown FK	(E154)
Brown HT	(E155)
Carotenes	(E160a)
Cochineal	(E120)
Erythrosine	(E127)
Green S	E142)
Indigotine, Indigo carmine	(E132)
Patent Blue V	(E131)
Ponceau 4R, Cochineal Red A, Brilliant Scarlet 4R	(E124)
Quinoline yellow	(E104)
Red 2G	E128)
Sunset Yellow FCF / Orange Yellow S	(E110)
Tartrazine	(E102)
Yellow 2G	(E107)

Preservatives

Benzoic acid	(E210)
Calcium benzoate	(E213)
Calcium hydrogen sulphite	(E227)
Calcium propionate	(E282)
Calcium sulphite	(E226)
Ethyl p-hydroxybenzoate	(E214)
Methyl p-hydroxybenzoate	(E218)
Potassium benzoate	(E212)
Potassium hydrogen sulphite	(E228)
Potassium metabisulphite	(E224)
Propyl p-hydroxybenzoate	(E216)
Sodium benzoate	(E211)
Sodium ethyl p-hydroxybenzoate	(E215)
Sodium hydrogen sulphite	(E222)
Sodium metabisulphite	(E223)

Sodium methyl p-hydroxybenzoate .... (E219)
Sodium propyl p-hydroxybenzoate .... (E217)
Sodium sulphite .... (E221)
Sulphur dioxide .... (E220)

Antioxidants
Butylated hydroxytoluene (BHT) .... (E321)
Dodecyl gallate .... (E312)
Octyl gallate .... (E311)
Propyl gallate .... (E310)

Acidity regulators
Nicotinic acid, niacin, nicotinamide .... (E375)

Thickeners/stabilizers/emulsifiers
Acacia gum (gum arabic) .... (E414)
Carrageenan .... (E407)
Karaya gum .... (E416)
Polyoxyethylene (8) stearate .... (E430)
Tragacanth .... (E413)

Acidity regulator/improving agent/firming agent
Talc .... (E553b)

Glazing agents
Beeswax, white and yellow .... (E901)
Carnauba wax .... (E903)

'Safe' Additives

Finally, the following additives are generally regarded as unlikely to provoke an allergic response and so are thought to be 'safe':

Agar .... (E406)
Alginic acid .... (E400)
Alpha-tocopherol .... (E307)
Aluminium silicate (Kaolin) .... (E559)
Ammonia caramel .... (E150c)
Annatto, bixin, norbixin .... (E160b)
Ascorbic acid .... (E300)
Beetroot Red, betanin .... (E162)

Chapter Six

More Fibre and Fluid

Two of the most important dietary changes you can make are to increase the amount of fibre and water you consume. Both are deficient in the average Western diet, yet at optimum levels they can have a profound effect on IBS symptoms. A healthy diet should contain at least 25 g of fibre (some experts recommend 35 g). This is more than the 10–15 g normally consumed in the West. In Africa and Asia, the daily average is up to 80 g.

Fibre can only be really beneficial if you also have plenty of fluids. The average adult body is over 60 per cent (nearly two-thirds) water. This level is quickly depleted unless replaced regularly. We lose at least 1.5 litres (over $2^{1}/_{2}$ pints) of water in the breath, sweat and faeces, quite apart from the amount we lose when urinating. This loss more than doubles in hot weather or when exercising.

Because of the dehydrating effect of modern central heating and air conditioning, most people live in unnaturally arid conditions. Dehydration is compounded by the amount of tea, coffee and alcohol the average person consumes. These drinks are diuretics – they cause you to urinate more, so you expel more fluid than you take in.

Fantastic Fibre
Increasing the amount of fibre in the diet can be beneficial to both constipation-dependent and diarrhoea-dependent IBS sufferers. This may seem contradictory, as fibre is mainly thought of as being helpful to those who have difficulty passing stools. In the case of diarrhoea sufferers, it would seem that fibre is the last thing they need. Fibre, however, is highly efficient at absorbing water – including the excess liquid in the bowel – and adding bulk to waste matter, so helping to regulate the passage of waste through the bowel. This is just as important for D-IBS sufferers as it is for those suffering from constipation, as it helps to reduce the sense of urgency and the need to rush to the toilet. In addition, the extra bulk keeps the bowel slightly distended, and this may help prevent the muscle spasms responsible for many of the IBS symptoms.

Types of Fibre
There are two main forms of fibre, soluble and insoluble, and both can aid IBS. Fibre cannot be broken down by digestive enzymes (although some forms can be digested by gut bacteria; see Chapter Three). Soluble and

insoluble fibre have a remarkable capacity to absorb water, swelling up to fifteen times in size. This keeps stools soft and malleable and provides the bulk needed to push the waste along by muscular action. As the names suggest, the main difference between the two is that soluble fibres dissolve in water and turn into gels (so are known as 'gel-forming fibres'), but insoluble fibres do not.

Soluble Fibre
Soluble fibre is further subdivided into two main types: mucilage, found in pulses, such as peas, beans and lentils, and pectins, found mainly in fruit and some vegetables. Mucilage is a highly efficient lubricant, too, and so eases the passage of waste matter through the bowel, as well as soothing the gut lining.

Insoluble Fibre
Insoluble fibre, or cellulose, is found in unprocessed cereals, fibrous vegetables and unpeeled fruits, such as apricots. The best-known insoluble fibre, bran, comes from the outer husk of wheat grains, which is retained in wholewheat products but removed in the refining process that produces white flour. Bran is sold separately as a fibre supplement, to be sprinkled on breakfast cereals, for example, or added as thickening to soups, stews and casseroles.

Soluble Fibre and Heart Disease
Soluble fibre also binds with cholesterol, a component of bile, which is produced by the liver and secreted into the digestive tract to help break down dietary fats. By locking on to the cholesterol in the gut, soluble fibre prevents its reabsorption, allowing it to be carried out with the waste. The liver uses the cholesterol in the bloodstream to make up the shortfall, which reduces the overall blood level. This helps prevent cardiovascular disease. Brands of cholesterol-lowering margarine work this way.

Without adequate dietary levels of soluble fibre (and mono-unsaturated fats, such as olive oil, which have a similar effect), cholesterol is deposited on the walls of blood vessels as fatty plaques. These plaques can build up and block a major blood vessel, for example in the heart, or break off and cause a blockage elsewhere, such as in the brain leading to heart attack and stroke.

Dual-fibre Foods
Some foods contain soluble and insoluble fibre, giving the best of both worlds. They include wholegrains, pulses, nuts, seeds, tuberous vegetables, and fruits with edible peel, such as cherries, plums, peaches

and apricots. The insoluble fibre is in the outer covering and the soluble fibre is incorporated into the bulk of the food. For example, a grain of wheat or rice contains an outer husk (bran) and a starchy interior containing soluble fibre. Potatoes contain insoluble fibre in their peel. It follows from this that you can regulate your intake of insoluble fibre by removing or consuming edible skin/peel, such as potato jackets or apple skin, as a way of fine-tuning your fibre intake.

Adding Fibre to the Diet

The best way to increase your fibre intake is to eat more fruit, vegetables, pulses and wholegrains. Brown rice, corn and oats tend to be well tolerated by IBS sufferers. Fruit and vegetables are particularly beneficial because of their high soluble fibre content. Their soothing, lubricating and bulk-forming properties ease muscle spasms and abdominal pain and promote regular bowel function.

More care should be taken when increasing the insoluble fibre content of the diet. Bran and pulses, for example, are often poorly tolerated in IBS sufferers, sometimes causing abdominal pain, bloating and flatulence without improving bowel habit. It is important to increase your insoluble fibre intake gradually, allowing the body time to cope with the change. Most people adjust within a few weeks, if not sooner.

If you've been used to a relatively low-fibre diet you may find that a sudden increase in insoluble fibre, such as bran, makes symptoms worse. Rather than making a dramatic switch from processed cereals, such as white rice, white flour and white pasta, to wholegrain types, one approach is to mix the two together. Start with a smaller percentage of wholegrain types and slowly increase the ratio as your digestion adapts to the change. This should ensure a slow but steady improvement in symptoms, rather than an initial deterioration, as may happen with a total switch to a high-fibre diet.

You could cook together brown and white rice, or wholemeal and white pasta (in the ratio of 1:3 wholegrain : processed to start with). Remember to allow a slightly longer cooking time to allow for the wholegrain portion. Similarly with bread, eat half a slice of wholemeal bread for every slice of white bread. As you find you can tolerate wholegrains, you can increase the amount eaten at each meal.

Electric breadmakers have made home baking much easier. One advantage they offer – as well as delicious fresh-baked bread whenever you want it – is that you can customize the recipe by increasing the fibre content to a level you can happily tolerate. In Chapter Nine there is a recipe for a mixed-grain loaf made in a breadmaker, containing about one-third wholemeal flour. Other recipes in that chapter contain a good proportion of fibre in a form most IBS sufferers should be able to tolerate.

Warning

When increasing the fibre content of your diet, and especially if using fibre supplements, make sure you increase your fluid intake accordingly. Without sufficient fluid, fibre becomes dangerously compacted in the bowel, a condition that requires medical aid and can be life-threatening.

Fibre Supplements

You can also take fibre as a supplement, usually in powder or pill form. This works the same way as the integral fibre in food. For some people, it is easier to increase dietary fibre using supplements than by increasing their intake of fruit and vegetables. Ideally, though, most fibre in the diet should come from natural sources.

Fibre supplements have the same advantages and drawbacks as high-fibre foods. Soluble fibre supplements are preferable, because of their gentle soothing and lubricating effect. Insoluble fibre supplements can trigger spasms and so may cause pain and constipation in some people. If using fibre supplements, take care to follow the instructions on the packet, and, in particular, drink a large glass of water with the supplement and have plenty of fluids throughout the day (see warning above).

As with high-fibre foods, increase your intake of fibre supplements slowly. For example, in the case of fibre powders, start with a half to one teaspoonful taken twice daily, and slowly, over the coming days and weeks, increase your intake to two tablespoons (or the maximum stipulated on the packet), or less than this if you find an optimum level that works best for you. Reduce your intake if symptoms start to worsen. Similarly with fibre supplements in pill form, start with one or two pills per day and increase the number to the recommended maximum, or fewer if you prefer.

If one type of fibre supplement seems to trigger IBS symptoms, it may be because you are sensitive to one of the ingredients, apart from the fibre. So always check the label. For example, some sugar-free brands contain artificial sweeteners such as aspartame (see Chapter Five) that some sufferers cannot tolerate. Orange-flavoured types include citric acid, another potentially problematic substance. Rather than abandon the notion of supplements, you could simply try a different brand.

Wonderful Water

Water is a vital but under-regarded component of a healthy diet. It makes good general health sense to drink plenty of water each day, but it is absolutely essential if you plan to increase the fibre content of your diet.

Insoluble fibre in particular is highly absorbent and can form a solid mass that the bowel cannot shift, unless you ensure that you drink plenty of fluids with – and especially after – your meals.

The average adult should drink at least 2 litres (3½pints) of water a day. This level should be increased during hot weather, or when exercising, or if you are pregnant or breastfeeding. If you are ill, and especially if you have been vomiting or are suffering from diarrhoea, it is important to increase your fluid intake accordingly. However, aim to limit your intake of tea, coffee and alcohol throughout the day.

Don't wait until you feel thirsty to have a drink because thirst is not a good indicator of your fluid level. A better guide is your urine, which should be pale or straw-coloured. A dark amber colour indicates that your fluid level is low and urgently needs topping up. Pure water, whether bottled, boiled or tap, is the simplest form of drink, but some may find it unpalatable or just boring. One way to pep up a glass of water is to flavour it with lemon or lime juice, or a sprig of mint or other herbs.

You could also try herbal teas, and fruit and vegetable juices. But bear in mind that some herbal teas have a high acid content that can erode tooth enamel if consumed too often. Following a herbal drink with a small piece of cheese can neutralize the acidity.

Fruit juices are usually high in sugar, which can cause tooth decay and may encourage overgrowth of the pathogenic yeast *Candida albicans* (see Chapter Four), so it is a good idea to dilute fruit juices and, where possible, consume them only at meal times. This also helps to avoid the rapid energy swings that can be associated with a high sugar intake. Much of your daily fluid intake comes from the food you eat. So an easy way to increase your daily liquid consumption is to eat more fruit and vegetables that have a high water content, such as pears, apples, grapes and tomatoes.

Chapter Seven

Star Foods for IBS

In general, a diet that is high in fruit, vegetables and wholegrain cereals, and low in sugar and fat, will benefit everyone. However, there are special foods that are of particular value to IBS sufferers. For example, apricots are especially high in fibre, which aids the passage of waste through the bowel.

Some fruits and vegetables contain oligosaccharides, the special form of fibre that supports the beneficial bacteria in the gut, principally Bifidobacteria and *Lactobacillus* (see Chapter Three). Other foods offer a delicious and nutritious alternative to problem items such as dairy products and wheat that can exacerbate IBS symptoms in some sufferers. Some foods, such as soya, satisfy several requirements. Garlic contains sulphur compounds and oils with anti-microbial effects, selectively targeting harmful microbes but, amazingly, leaving beneficial bacteria unaffected.

Many foods that contain prebiotic oligosaccharides, such as bananas, garlic, onions, leeks, peas and wheat, are already staples in the average diet. Other foods, such as artichoke, asparagus, barley, oats and olives, are eaten less often, and some foods, such as chicory, rarely feature on the shopping list. Yet all these foods can make delicious additions to the menu.

It has been estimated that to maintain a healthy population of beneficial gut bacteria we need to consume at least 5 g of oligosaccharides every day. But the modern diet probably contains as little as 3 g. So, to try to redress the balance, aim to include some of the following foods in your diet on a regular basis. Chicory is high in FOS; it is an acquired taste but with the right preparation can add a distinctive flavour to a recipe.

Health-giving Properties

The foods described in this chapter do not represent all the products that can be beneficial in the management of IBS. They have been chosen mainly as some of the best examples. Many of these foods have a wide range of health-giving properties. Members of the onion family, for example, contain sulphur compounds that have an anti-microbial action. The oil in coconut (and especially its active ingredient, lauric acid) is effective against candida.

Oats and barley are an important source of iron and soluble fibre and make a well-tolerated alternative to wheat products. Soya is low in fat –

especially saturated fat – but high in protein, and so makes a good substitute for fatty cuts of meat. Beans, peas, lentils and other pulses are high in fibre, and brown rice, corn, quinoa and wild rice are usually better tolerated by IBS sufferers than wheat.

Almonds (*Prunus dulcis*)
Almonds have the highest fibre content of any nut and so can play an important part in alleviating IBS symptoms. They contain many other health benefits, too. They are high in monounsaturated fat, which can help reduce blood cholesterol levels, and are a rich source of the antioxidant nutrient vitamin E, which protects against heart disease. They are also one of the best non-dairy sources of calcium, for strong bones and teeth. A very versatile nut, almonds can be chopped and added to breakfast cereals, served with salads, baked in cakes or added to casseroles. They can also be toasted – simply heat them gently in a pan for a few minutes. Choose unblanched almonds, where possible, ideally freshly shelled, as these have the highest nutrient levels.

Apricots (*Prunus armenia*)
Apricots are high in soluble and insoluble fibre, which makes them ideal for IBS sufferers. They are one of the best sources of beta-carotene, an important antioxidant which can help prevent heart disease and cancer. As a general rule, the brighter the colour the higher the beta-carotene content (that holds true for most brightly coloured fruits). Beta-carotene is converted to vitamin A in the body, which is important for good eyesight. Apricots contain high levels of potassium, which helps prevent high blood pressure, and iron, which guards against anaemia. Apricots also contain boron, which aids calcium absorption and so helps prevent osteoporosis.

Dried apricots have especially high levels of fibre, beta-carotene, potassium and iron. Just a handful of apricots (around 40 g) supplies 20 per cent of an adult's recommended daily potassium intake, and 10 per cent of a woman's daily iron needs. But most dried apricots also contain sulphur, which can trigger IBS symptoms in some sufferers. Sulphur-free dried apricots are available from health food stores. Apricots are delicious and versatile fruits, eaten fresh, on their own or mixed with other fruits in desserts and salads, or steamed, baked or dried. Chopped and added to breakfast cereals such as muesli or porridge, they offer a delicious and nutritious start to the day.

Asparagus (*Asparagus officinalis*)
Asparagus, which is a member of the lily family, has been a popular vegetable since Elizabethan times. It contains high levels of vitamins C and

E, folate (folic acid) and minerals including potassium, calcium and iron. Yet it is remarkably low in calories. The edible parts are long, slender green spears, topped by tiny bunches of tightly folded purple leaves. The tips and upper parts are tender, but the stems become tougher towards the base.

Asparagus is often enjoyed as a starter, by simply eating the succulent tips and upper stems (usually dipped in sauce), and leaving the tougher lower stem portions behind. The lower sections need not be wasted, however. They can be cut off before serving, peeled and stored for a short time to be added to soups, stews and casseroles, to provide extra flavour and nutrients, where the longer cooking time softens them. The delicate tips cook faster than the stems, so asparagus is often tied in a bundle and cooked standing upright. Asparagus can also be grilled, which imparts a lovely smoky flavour. Brush with olive oil and turn frequently.

Bananas (*Musa cavendishii*)
In addition to oligosaccharides, bananas are rich in micro-nutrients, including vitamins C, B3, B5 and B6, and the mineral potassium, which counterbalances sodium (salt) in the diet and so helps maintain healthy blood pressure. They provide a good form of easily obtainable energy. More importantly, this energy is released at a sustainable rate – unlike the sugar 'rush' (followed by the equally rapid energy slump) you get from sweets and biscuits. Bananas also contain a natural antacid that helps relieve heartburn.

Bananas are both delicious and versatile, and so easy to include in the diet. They can be chopped up and added to breakfast cereal to stock up your energy levels for the day ahead. They can be eaten between meals to tide you over mid-morning/mid-afternoon fatigue. And they can be incorporated into a wide range of puddings (or eaten on their own with custard). Finally, bananas can be blended with other fruit to make a nutritious 'smoothie' drink (see recipes, Chapter Nine).

Barley (*Hordeum sp.*)
Barley is mainly associated with the brewing industry and is not a major component of the average diet today, which is a great shame. Like other wholegrains, barley is a good source of B vitamins and minerals such as iron and zinc. It is best to eat the wholegrain form, pot barley, which still contains all the important nutrients, rather than heavily processed pearl barley grains. You can also buy whole hulled barley, in which only the outer husk is removed, or coarsely ground barley meal.

In addition to the bacteria-boosting oligosaccharides it contains, barley is high in all forms of fibre – five or six times more than most wholegrains – and especially soluble forms. This form of fibre brings all sorts of health benefits, including lowering blood cholesterol levels, so helping to guard against heart disease, regulating blood sugar levels, which reduces the risk of developing type II (adult onset) diabetes, and offering some protection against various forms of cancer, especially of the breast and colon. There are quick-cooking barley products available that can be used as a delicious alternative to rice and pasta. You can also add barley to stews, casseroles and hotpots.

Brown rice (*Oryza sativa*)

Rice, like all carbohydrates, is a good source of energy and makes a delicious alternative to bread and potatoes in the diet. However, white rice, the form generally consumed in the West, has been processed to remove the husk, which contains most of the vitamins and minerals and all of the fibre. Therefore switching to brown rice not only helps to boost the fibre content of your diet, but also raises the level of other important nutrients, such as vitamins B1 and B3, iron, magnesium and zinc.

Many IBS sufferers find that the fibre found in brown rice is less problematic than cereal-based fibre, such as bran. Rice also makes a gluten-free alternative to wheat flour in rice bread and rice cakes, and rice milk is a good substitute for cow's milk.

Buckwheat (*Fagopyrum sp.*)

Buckwheat is a staple food crop in parts of Russia, where it is always left unrefined to retain all its fibre and micro-nutrient content. It is high in selenium, an antioxidant mineral that has anti-ageing effects and also helps prevent heart disease and cancer, vitamin A, which is important for eyesight and helps boost the immune system, vitamin B for energy and a healthy nervous system, and the antioxidant vitamin E. Buckwheat is also a rich source of lysine, an essential amino acid not found in most plant sources of protein, and so a useful addition to the diet for vegans.

Buckwheat is not actually related to wheat (it is a member of the rhubarb family) and so does not contain gluten, which makes it a problem-free alternative for those who are sensitive to wheat-based products. It has a pleasantly nutty flavour and can be served as a cereal or a side dish, or added to soups, stews and casseroles.

Chicory (*Cichorium intybus*)

Chicory is a member of the lettuce family. There are different forms: loose-leafed types, compact and spear-shaped types, and broad-leafed radicchio types. It has other names including endive, Belgian endive, Brussels chicory and witloof (white leaf). It is the richest known edible source of the oligosaccharide FOS, and contains many important nutrients, including vitamins C, E and folate (the plant form of folic acid, a member of the B complex), the minerals iron and potassium, and the antioxidant carotene.

Chicory can be baked, braised, steamed or served raw in salads. It has a tangy, bitter flavour that makes it a useful accompaniment to rich and creamy meals. It can be served in a salad dressed with lemon juice, vinaigrette and seasoned olive oil, and goes well with citrus fruits, such as orange, or a creamy cheese. To help reduce the bitterness, simply cut each spear (or 'chicon', as it is known) in half and remove the central core, which is the strongest-flavoured part.

Coconut (*Cocos nucifera*)

Coconut is not normally associated with therapeutic foods. In part this is because it is high in saturated fat, which should be kept to a minimum in the diet. Yet coconut oil has beneficial qualities too. It protects against a wide range of infections and infestations of the digestive tract, including the bacteria *Helicobacter pylori*, *Staphylococcus aureus*, *Chlamydia trachomatis*, *Streptococcus sp.*, the fungi *Candida albicans* and *Tinea sp.*, and the single-celled parasite *Giardia lamblia*. It also has antiviral properties, and can enhance the effectiveness of antibiotics and other drugs. Coconut has many culinary uses in cakes and desserts, and also in savoury dishes such as Thai curries.

Corn (*Zea mays*)

Health experts are constantly exhorting us to increase our consumption of wholegrain foods in preference to processed cereals (such as white flour) and to vary the types of grain in the diet. This way, we increase our fibre intake and benefit from all the micro-nutrients which wholegrains provide. Corn is a good example. This versatile cereal is packed with fibre – including oligosaccharides – and contains important amounts of B vitamins and the mineral iron.

Also known as maize, corn is produced in many forms: corn on the cob, polenta, popcorn, sweetcorn and – in the United States – grits. Boiled (or tinned), it can be added to salads and pizza toppings, included in sandwich fillings, or served up as an extra vegetable with meat, fish and vegetarian dishes. As an unrefined flour – ground cornmeal – it retains the all-important fibre and other nutrients, and can be used in place of wheat in many dishes. For example, it can be made into quick breads, puddings and cakes.

Cranberry (*Vaccinium macrocarpon*)

There are two principal species of cranberry, the smaller European form and the larger North American one. The latter is mainly used in the popular fruit juice. Native North Americans were aware of cranberry's medicinal properties long before European settlers discovered it, using it to treat various digestive ailments. It is rich in antioxidants, including vitamin C (100 ml of cranberry juice contains 50 per cent of the recommended daily allowance), and proanthocyanidins. This means it can aid cardiovascular health and help protect against cancer. Studies have shown that it is as effective as red wine at regulating blood cholesterol levels. Cranberry juice is a well-proven treatment for urinary tract infections. It stops harmful bacteria sticking to the bladder wall, allowing them to be flushed away in the urine. It is thought that it may fulfil a similar function in the bowel. It may also reduce the risk of gum disease and stomach ulcers. Cranberry's mix of sweet and tangy flavours combines well with other berries, in a summer pudding for example, or it can be blended with bananas, pears and other fruits in a smoothie.

Garlic (*Allium sativum*)
Garlic has an ancient history, and is valued for both its culinary and therapeutic uses. It is one of the most powerful medicinal plants of all, with a wide range of effects. A member of the onion family, garlic contains vitamin B6 and a wealth of minerals including iron, magnesium, potassium and zinc. It is also rich in antioxidant plant chemicals, called flavonoids, and volatile oils, such as allicin. Garlic oil has many therapeutic effects. For example, it can reduce the risk of heart disease by thinning the blood and lowering blood cholesterol levels. Garlic oil combats pathogenic fungi and bacteria – including antibiotic-resistant strains – but is particularly effective against *Candida albicans, Salmonella, Helicobacter pylori, Streptococcus, Vibrio metchnikovii, Vibrio parahaemolyticus* and *Brucella*. The peeled cloves (crushed, chopped or whole) contain oligosaccharides, which promote the growth of beneficial bacteria.

Garlic is a versatile food that complements any savoury dish. It can be finely chopped and mixed into a dressing, sprinkled over salads, or added to casseroles and stews (add near the end of cooking to preserve its active ingredients).

Jerusalem artichokes (*Helianthus tuberosus*)
Despite its name, Jerusalem artichoke is not related to the globe artichoke, which is a member of the thistle family. It is a form of sunflower. Jerusalem is merely a mishearing of girasole, the Italian word for sunflower. Jerusalem artichokes have edible potato-like tubers that are high in soluble and insoluble fibre and contain useful amounts of micro-nutrients, including B and C vitamins, and the minerals potassium, calcium and iron. They have a

starchy consistency and a nutty flavour. An easy way to use them is to cut them up and cook them with chopped potatoes until both are tender. Mash them together, with a tablespoon or two of good-quality margarine and a little soya milk. Add chopped parsley or other herbs and season to taste.

Leeks (*Allium porrum*)
Leeks have the same active ingredients, such as volatile oils – including sulphur compounds – that give onions their pungent aroma. However, they are present in leeks (and chives) in smaller amounts. This means that leeks may not offer the same level of health benefits, but will be more easily tolerated by those who are sensitive to other members of the onion family. Leeks also contain reasonable levels of oligosaccharides and other fibres, plus vitamins B1, C, E and folate, and the mineral iron.

To obtain maximum benefit from all the nutrients, leeks are best served raw, for example in salads, or only lightly cooked. Leeks are especially delicious blended into soups. They can also be added to casseroles, stews and hotpots or simply served as an additional vegetable with most meat, fish and vegetarian dishes.

Linseed (*Linum usitatissimum*)
Also known as flaxseed, linseed is a highly nutritious food that is rich in vitamin E, iron, zinc and omega-3 and omega-6 fatty acids. It contains both soluble and insoluble fibre and so is highly beneficial for managing IBS symptoms. There is also evidence that it may have a prebiotic effect, encouraging the growth of friendly gut bacteria.

Linseed can be used in many different ways. It can be added to soups and stews, ground up and mixed with breakfast cereals and flour, or sprinkled over meals. It also makes a simple laxative: take 1–2 tsp of ground linseed with up to 250 ml ($\frac{1}{2}$ pint) water each day.

Millet (*Panicum miliaceum*)
Millet is not widely eaten in the West, and yet is a good source of protein, vitamins and minerals and is well tolerated by those sensitive to wheat. Also known as sorghum, it is a staple food crop in many parts of the world, including southern Europe, Asia and North Africa, where it is ground to a flour and used to make bread and other baked foods. It can also be added to soups, stews and casseroles.

Oats (*Avena sativa*)
Like all cereals, oats are an important source of energy and protein. They are also rich in soluble fibre and so help lower blood cholesterol and reduce the

risk of heart disease and stroke. Also important, in the context of IBS, they contain oligosaccharides and are often well tolerated – even in those sensitive to wheat products. (However, as they contain gluten they may not be suitable for those with coeliac disease; see Chapter Twelve.) Oats are a good source of B and E vitamins, and are high in iron, as well as containing magnesium, potassium, selenium and zinc. It is easy to increase your daily consumption of oats. Oat-rich porridge and muesli provide an energy-packed start to the day, and oats can be baked into biscuits, or turned into a delicious fruit crumble dessert.

Olives (*Olea europaea*)
Olive oil is now the standard oil for cooking and salad dressing. But the oil lacks the important bacteria-boosting oligosaccharides found in the fruit itself. Olives are high in fat, and so should be eaten sparingly. However, this is the healthy monounsaturated form of fat that actually helps lower blood cholesterol levels and guards against heart disease and strokes. Olives, whether stuffed, stoned or natural, are a popular hors d'oeuvre and accompaniment to pizza, salads and kebabs. They can also be added to baked dishes and stir-fries to provide additional nutrients – and a Mediterranean touch.

Onions (*Allium sepa*)
The onion family is very large, and includes shallots, chives and spring onions (as well as garlic and leeks – see above). All members of the family contain oligosaccharides plus vitamins, such as B1 and B6, and important plant chemicals, including sulphur compounds, which help lower blood pressure and blood cholesterol, and fight infection. Like leeks, chives have low levels of sulphur compounds and so are less pungent than other members. They can be chopped into egg dishes and salads or added as a garnish.

Onions have many culinary uses and so there is no excuse not to eat them on a regular basis. The sulphur compounds that give raw onions their sharp, tangy flavour help enliven salads, and complement cheese and meat dishes. The tang is lost when cooked, but onions retain a rich flavour that gives body to soups, stews, casseroles and stir-fries.

Pears (*Pyrus communis*)
Like many fruits, pears are a good source of soluble fibre, in the form of pectin, but they are also high in insoluble fibre (around 3 g per pear, on average), which makes them an ideal food for promoting bowel health. They are also a good source of vitamin C and potassium. They have the distinction of being one of the few foods not associated with any allergies,

and so can safely be included in an elimination diet.

Peas (*Pisum sativum*)

Like all pulses, peas provide a good supply of vegetable protein and therefore are important to vegetarians and vegans, or indeed anyone who wants to reduce their meat consumption. Peas are also high in energy, but as this is combined with fibre they are digested slowly, ensuring a steady, controllable rise in blood sugar levels. They are one of the richest natural sources of vitamin B1, and contain useful amounts of vitamin C, folate (folic acid), the minerals calcium and iron and phytochemicals.

Peas are a standard 'second vegetable' in many traditional meals and so easily disregarded. Yet they come in many different varieties, including mangetout and sugar snap, of which both pods and peas are eaten, and minted garden and tinned marrowfat, with their own unique flavours and culinary uses. Mangetout and sugar snap are delicious in stir-fries and can also be added to salads to give variety.

Quinoa (*Chenopodium quinoa*)

Quinoa is the fruit of a South American herb and has long been prized as a valuable source of energy for those working at high altitudes in the Andes. It is rich in good-quality protein (accounting for 16 per cent of its calories – four times as much as corn) containing all eight essential amino acids, and so makes an important contribution to the diet for non-meat eaters. It is also a good source of essential fatty acids, vitamins, including B complex and E, and the minerals calcium, iron and potassium.

Quinoa is generally treated as a grain, rather than a fruit, but is unusual in having more essential fats than fruit, and more protein than grains. It has a mild flavour and can be served as an accompaniment to meat, fish and vegetable dishes or added to stews, casseroles and breakfast cereals. It makes a good alternative to rice and can be cooked in much the same way, simply add twice as much water as quinoa, bring to the boil and simmer for 15 minutes, or until all the water has been absorbed.

Soya beans (*Glycine max*)

Soya also contains another source of oligosaccharides. However, this form, known as xylooligosacharides, is not thought to be quite as effective at boosting levels of friendly bacteria as the other forms – fructo- and galacto-oligosaccharides (see Chapter Three). But soya has other beneficial properties that make up for these shortcomings. It is a rich source of protein, but low in saturated fat and so is a healthy alternative to meat. It is packed with vital micro-nutrients, including B and E vitamins, and minerals such as calcium, iron, selenium and zinc.

Soya does not have much flavour itself, but it can be converted into numerous different forms to be used as an alternative to animal products. For example, textured soya protein can be used in place of meat in many dishes. Tempeh and tofu are types of fermented beancurd, made in a process involving live bacteria, rather like cheese-making. They can be chopped, sliced or crumbled and then flavoured and added to a wide range of dishes. Soya is also available as a flour.

Soya milk, usually fortified with extra calcium, is a good dairy milk substitute. It is often sweetened with apple juice to make it more palatable. It is a boon to those who are sensitive to milk (and especially lactose). Live soya yoghurt is available for those who cannot tolerate milk-based yoghurt.

Wild rice (*Zizania aquatica*)
This is the seed of a species of aquatic grass that was the staple food of many native North American tribes but is now becoming increasingly popular in Europe. It is a good source of protein and vitamins, and can be cooked like rice and served to accompany meat, fish and vegetable dishes or mixed with brown rice to add variety and extra nutritional value to a meal.

Chapter Eight

Medicinal Herbs and Spices

Herbs, spices and plant oils normally associated with the kitchen garden often have medicinal properties that are particularly helpful for IBS sufferers. Some contain natural compounds that combat pathogenic organisms known, or believed, to trigger IBS. Among the oils receiving the most intensive study for their antifungal, anti-parasitic and anti-bacterial properties are, in addition to garlic oil (see Chapter Seven), cinnamon oil, clove oil, ginger oil, oregano oil and rosemary oil. Cinnamon and oregano are especially useful against the infectious yeast *Candida albicans* (see Chapter Four).

Therapeutic Effects

Antispasmodic herbs soothe the muscular spasms in the bowel wall associated with abdominal pain, diarrhoea and constipation. Carminative herbs release trapped wind and relieve bloating, flatulence and indigestion. Some herbs, known as demulcents and emollients, contain substances such as pectin and mucilage that soothe and lubricate the gut. Other herbs are natural sedatives and so have calming and mood-enhancing properties, alleviating IBS symptoms indirectly by easing stress, anxiety and depression.

Herbs are best used fresh, so if you find any herbs particularly beneficial you might consider growing them in the garden, or in a pot on the windowsill. A good herb nursery or specialist supplier can advise.

How They Are Used

Many of the herbs and spices listed here have both culinary and medicinal uses. They can be used to pep up soups, stews and casseroles and to enliven meat, fish and vegetable dishes, or added to cakes and desserts. The great advantage of herbal flavouring is that it does not greatly increase the calorific content of a meal, as sugar does, or trigger health problems (such as raised blood pressure and stroke) as salt can.

Some herbs are only used for their therapeutic properties. These are best taken as a soothing drink. Herbs that can be highly beneficial for IBS symptoms include agrimony, catmint, chamomile, fennel, ginger, lemon balm and peppermint. Herbal remedies are usually taken as an infusion, like tea. Simply put one or two teaspoons of the chopped leaves (or finely chopped root, in the case of ginger) in a tea pot and pour boiling water over. Leave to infuse for 5–10 minutes. Strain the mixture into a cup, add sugar or honey to taste and allow to cool before drinking. You can drink up to four cups a day, as required. You can also mix them together, for example combining one teaspoon each of the chopped leaves of agrimony, chamomile and lemon balm in the pot.

Dill and fennel seeds are best served as a decoction. Add one tablespoon of whole dill seeds or two teaspoons of whole fennel seeds to 300 ml ($\frac{1}{2}$pt) of water in a small saucepan, bring to the boil and simmer for 10 minutes. Add sugar or honey to taste and allow to cool before drinking.

Caution: Always obtain herbs and herbal remedies from established suppliers only. If you are pregnant, or suffering from high blood pressure, heart, kidney or liver disease, or other serious disorder, check with a doctor before taking herbal preparations.

Star Herbs and Spices

The following herbs and spices have proven or well-established therapeutic properties that may be beneficial for IBS sufferers.

Agrimony (*Agrimonia eupatoria*)

Agrimony is a member of the rose family. Agrimony leaves, stems and flowers have a long history of use in herbal medicine, both internally, taken as an infusion or used as a gargle, and externally as a compress. Agrimony contains volatile oils such as borneol acetate that act as an antispasmodic to ease cramping, a carminative to ease bloating and flatulence, an anti-inflammatory to ease allergic reactions, and an astringent to alleviate diarrhoea. It may not be suitable for constipation sufferers, however. Agrimony is easy to grow and its leaves can be picked when needed to use in an infusion.

Catmint (*Nepeta cataria*)

Also known as catnip, catmint leaves and flowering tops contain volatile oils that help to alleviate bloating, spasms, cramping, flatulence, diarrhoea and indigestion, and promote regular bowel movement. They can be chopped finely and added to sauces and stews to give a mint-like flavouring, or used in an infusion. Catmint can be grown as a garden plant (but beware of cats, which find it irresistible). Pick young leaves for flavouring, or use fresh or dried leaves for an infusion.

Chamomile (*Matricaria recutita*)

Chamomile makes a delicious and soothing infusion. Chamomile flowers contain coumarins, salicylic acid (a component of aspirin) and mucilage to soothe the bowel and prevent muscle spasms, so helping to ease pain, relieve nervous indigestion, alleviate diarrhoea or constipation and release trapped wind. Chamomile can also calm nerves and aid restful sleep. The flowers are best picked when first fully open.

Chicory (*Cichorium intybus*)

Chicory makes a useful vegetable (see Chapter Seven) as it contains the prebiotic fibre that promotes healthy gut bacteria, such as *Bifidobacterium*. (see Chapter Seven) However, the leaves can be infused to make a tea that aids digestion, and the root can be roasted and ground to make a caffeine-free coffee substitute.

Cinnamon (*Cinnamon zeylanicum*)

As well as being a popular dessert spice, cinnamon has a long history as a medicinal herb. Traditionally it was used to treat colic, diarrhoea, dyspepsia and flatulence. The principal active ingredient of cinnamon oil is cinnamaldehyde, which gives the spice its characteristic smell and flavour. The oil has been shown to inhibit a wide range of pathogenic microbes including *Escherichia coli*, *Helicobacter pylori* (which causes stomach ulcers), *Klebsiella, Listeria* and *Salmonella*, and the fungi *Aspergillus flavus*, *Aspergillus parasiticus*, *Candida albicans* and *Fusarium moniliforme*. Cinnamon oil was shown to be effective against not only the fungi themselves, but also the toxins they produce. In a study reported to the annual meeting of the Institute of Food Technologists in Chicago in 1999, just one teaspoon of cinnamon, added to an apple juice sample contaminated with one million *E. coli bacteria* wiped out 99.5 per cent of the pathogens.

Clove (*Eugenia aromatica*)

This pungent spice comes from the dried flower-bud of a tropical plant. Clove is another spice that has a long tradition of both culinary and therapeutic use, particularly in the treatment of diarrhoea, flatulence, indigestion and nausea. The principal active ingredient is eugenol, which makes up 90 per cent of the oil extract. In studies, clove has been shown to exert its most powerful inhibitory effect against the bacteria *Escherichia coli*, *Listeria monocytogenes* and *Salmonella enterica*, and the fungi *Aspergillus parasiticus*, *Aspergillus flavus*, *Aspergillus versicolor and Fusarium moniliforme*.

Dill (*Anethum graveolens*)

The leaves and seeds of dill, and the oil extracted from them, all have culinary uses. The leaves and seeds in particular are used in Scandinavian and Mediterranean recipes, and in egg, seafood and potato dishes, rice, soups and pickles. The seeds are also used in curry powder. Its therapeutic effects are well established, especially in alleviating abdominal ailments. Dill is the main ingredient in gripe water, a traditional remedy for infant digestive upsets. Dill has antispasmodic and carminative properties, easing muscular spasms, bloating and flatulence. The leaves can be used in an infusion and the seeds in a decoction.

Fennel (*Foeniculum vulgare*)

Fennel contains two principal and contrasting oils: bitter-tasting fenchone and sweet-tasting anethole. Depending on the proportions of these two oils, the leaves can be bitter or sweet, often tasting like anise. Leaves, roots, seeds and oil have culinary uses, especially in fish and vegetable dishes, and in salads (leaves). The flower stems can be eaten like celery. Fennel has antispasmodic and carminative properties, helping to alleviate spasms, bloating and flatulence. Fennel leaves (bruised or crushed) can be used in an infusion and the seeds and chopped root in a decoction.

Ginger (*Zingiber officinale*)

Ginger is a popular and versatile flavouring, used in oriental dishes, especially curries, and in biscuits, cakes, desserts and confectionery products. The principal active oil is zingiberole, which gives it its distinctive hot flavour. Ginger has long been recognized as a digestive tonic with both antispasmodic and carminative properties. It is particularly useful in the relief of abdominal pain, nausea and sickness because of its calming effect on the digestive tract. Its ability to combat harmful intestinal organisms is well known in Japan, where it is traditionally eaten with raw fish to counteract parasitic infestation. It is also thought to have antifungal properties, particularly against *Candida albicans*, and to inhibit pathogenic bacteria including *Campylobacter*, *Clostridium*, *Listeria* and *Staphylococcus*.

Lemon balm (*Melissa officinalis*)

Lemon balm is a multi-purpose herb: its leaves can be used to flavour savoury foods, such as sauces, soups, fish and poultry, and sweet dishes, including jams, ices and desserts. The leaves can also be eaten with salads or stirred into stews and casseroles. The principal therapeutic oils in lemon balm include citral, citronellol, eugenol and geraniol. These have antiviral properties and also contribute to its carminative and antispasmodic effects, alleviating bloating, spasms, cramping, flatulence and indigestion, and promoting regularity. Lemon balm is a mild sedative, helping to ease anxiety and stress. For the relief of symptoms, lemon balm is best taken as an infusion, either on its own or mixed with chamomile.

Oregano (*Oreganum vulgare*)
This spice is actually derived from the fresh or dried leaves of the herb wild marjoram and is added to a wide range of dishes. A closely related species, sweet marjoram (*Oreganum hortensis*) also has culinary and medicinal uses. Oregano oil contains the active ingredients carvacrol and thymol and has antiviral and antifungal properties, especially against *Candida albicans* and *Aspergillus* ochraceus. It is effective against antibiotic-resistant strains of *Escherichia coli*, *Listeria monocytogenes* and *Salmonella enterica* and has been used in the treatment of parasitic infestation by *Entamoeba histolica* and *Blastocystis hominis*. Remarkably, it also promotes the probiotic bacterium *Lactobacillus plantarum*, thought to be highly beneficial in IBS.

Peppermint (*Mentha X piperita*)
Peppermint is a very versatile herb, with a well-established place in the kitchen cupboard and the medicine cabinet. It is popularly used to flavour vegetables, especially peas and new potatoes, in desserts such as fruit salad, ice cream and sorbets, and in mint creams and other confectioneries. It contains numerous therapeutic oils, including carvone, cineol, limonene, menthol, menthone, pinene and thymol. Peppermint has carminative and antispasmodic properties to alleviate bloating, spasms, cramping, flatulence and indigestion, and to promote regular bowel movement. For relief of symptoms, it is most effective as an infusion or as a sweet.

Rosemary (*Rosmarinus officinalis*)
Rosemary has had a place in the culinary and therapeutic herb garden since the Middle Ages. It has many uses in herbal medicine, especially as an antispasmodic, to alleviate the cramping pain of IBS. Rosemary oil is now exciting renewed interest among medical researchers. In particular, carnosol, the main ingredient in rosemary oil, has powerful antioxidant effects, and may help counteract ageing, heart disease and cancer.

In addition, rosemary oil contains limonene and camphor, which contribute to the herb's distinctive scent, along with minerals and the antioxidant beta-carotene, which is converted to vitamin A in the body. Rosemary oil has powerful anti-bacterial properties, which are even more effective when combined with clove and cinnamon. This pungent herb has many culinary uses, including in roast lamb, baked fish, casseroles and potato dishes. Because of its tough, fibrous nature, it should be used finely chopped or removed before eating. Leaves and flowering tops are used in infusions and decoctions.

Chapter Nine

IBS Recipes

This collection of recipes can aid the management of IBS in several ways: some recipes offer nutritious alternatives to common foods known to aggravate symptoms, many contain soluble and/or insoluble fibre for healthy bowel function, others contain prebiotics, such as FOS (naturally or as a powder), or probiotic yoghurt to promote digestive health. Powdered FOS is available from many health food stores, by mail order or via the Internet. (If taking medication, check with your doctor before using FOS. Not to be used with drugs that are inhibited by pH lowering agents.)

The suggested foods are usually well tolerated by IBS sufferers. However, if you know or suspect any of the ingredients might trigger symptoms, try to find a suitable alternative. For example, in some recipes using butter will give a richer flavour and creamier texture, which some may prefer. But a good-quality margarine or vegetable oil will usually work just as well.

The metric and imperial measures given are not exact equivalents, so to ensure the proportions are correct please follow one or the other but do not mix the two.

For Breakfast

BANANA STARTER

This delicious high-energy drink will kick-start your day. The pears are high in soluble fibre and the banana is a rich natural source of FOS, which boosts the beneficial Bifidobacteria to aid a healthy digestive tract. To increase the soluble fibre, add 100 g (4 oz) of seasonal berries, such as blackberries, cherries, cranberries and blueberries, and/or 1 tsp of wheatgerm or sunflower seeds.

Ingredients
1 banana, peeled and sliced
2 pears, peeled, cored and chopped
150 ml (5 fl oz) live yoghurt

Method
Place all the ingredients in a food processor and blend to a smooth mixture.

Transfer to a suitable container and refrigerate. Serve chilled in two tall glasses

FRUIT SMOOTHIE
This delicious drink is packed with vitamins, natural enzymes and fibre for a morning tonic.

Ingredients
225 ml (8 fl oz) grape juice
225 ml (8 fl oz) orange juice
150 g (5 oz) mixed mango, melon and apricot, chopped
Crushed ice

Method
Place all the ingredients in a food processor and blend to a smooth mixture. Transfer to a suitable container and refrigerate. Serve chilled in two tall glasses.

NUTTY MUESLIi
A good, healthy breakfast makes a great start to the day. This high-energy recipe is rich in soluble fibre, and includes live yoghurt to promote digestive health. Soya milk is a good alternative to cow's milk for those who cannot tolerate dairy foods. Omit the sultanas, if preferred, and substitute sliced banana, chopped apricots or seasonal berries. If kept in an airtight container this muesli should last for up to a month.

Ingredients
125 g (5 oz) hazelnuts, crushed or coarsely chopped
125 g (5 oz) Brazil nuts, crushed or coarsely chopped
450 g (1 lb) rolled oats
8 tbsp honey
2 tbsp sunflower oil
sultanas (or other dried fruit of choice)

Method
Preheat the oven to 180° C/350° F/Gas 4. Mix together the nuts and oats, then stir in the honey and oil until well coated. Spread over two greased baking trays. Bake for 20–25 minutes, stirring occasionally until evenly browned. Leave to cool. Serve with soya milk, 1 tbsp live yoghurt and 2 tbsp sultanas, if appropriate. Makes about 1kg (2.2 lb).

ARTICHOKE AND LEEK SOUP

This dish features Jerusalem artichoke, leek and onion, which all contain the special type of prebiotic fibre known as FOS that promotes internal levels of friendly microbes. To prevent the chopped artichokes becoming discoloured, keep them under water until ready to use.

Ingredients
1 onion, peeled and chopped
450 g (1 lb) Jerusalem artichokes, peeled and sliced
2 leeks, sliced
1 clove garlic, crushed
2 tbsp olive oil (or 25 g/1 oz margarine or butter)
900 ml (30 fl oz) vegetable stock
300 ml (10 fl oz) soya milk (unsweetened)
salt and pepper

Method
Put the onion, artichoke and leek into a large pan and sauté until translucent. Add the vegetable stock and bring to the boil. Simmer for 30 to 40 minutes or until tender. Allow to cool and then transfer to a food processor and blend until smooth. Return to the pan and reheat, without boiling. Mix the cornflour to a paste with a little soya milk and stir into the soup. Continue stirring as you bring it to the boil. Add the rest of the soya milk and simmer for 10 minutes. Season to taste. Serve with crusty bread. Serves four.

LEEK AND POTATO SOUP
Leek contains the prebiotic fibre FOS and, like all members of the onion family, has important immune system-boosting properties. This recipe provides a warming, chunky soup that is ideal for cold days. It can also be blended for a smoother consistency.

Ingredients
4 leeks, chopped
50 g (2 oz) margarine (or butter)
4 medium potatoes, chopped
1.5 litres (3 pints) vegetable stock
salt and pepper to taste - and chopped chives, to garnish

Method
Place the margarine in a large pan, add the chopped leeks and sauté until translucent. Add the chopped potatoes and cook for a few minutes. Add the stock. Heat through and simmer for 30 minutes. Season to taste. Garnish with the chopped chives. Serve with crusty bread. Serves four.

COUNTRY LOAF

This delicious crusty loaf contains some soluble and insoluble fibre to promote regularity, but not so much that it will trigger symptoms. But avoid if you are highly sensitive to insoluble fibre. This recipe has worked in most breadmaking machines it has been tried in, but always follow the manufacturer's instructions on your breadmaker. The mixed grain/ sunflower seed bread mix is available from most large stores.

Ingredients
2 tbsp olive oil
450 ml (15 fl oz) lukewarm water
300 ml (11 oz) strong white bread flour
100 ml (4 oz) wholemeal bread flour
100 ml (4 oz) mixed grain (or sunflower seed) bread mix
½ level tsp sugar
½ level tsp dried yeast
½ level tsp salt
1 vitamin C tablet (200 mg), crushed

Method
Place all the ingredients in the breadmaker bin in the order given, taking care to avoid pouring the salt directly onto the yeast. Place the bin in the breadmaker and select the French bread setting (750 g size) and switch on. When baked, turn out onto a wire cooling rack and leave to cool for 1 hour.

For Starters

STEAMED ASPARAGUS

Asparagus is another good source of FOS, to feed and encourage beneficial bacteria. The easiest and healthiest way to cook them is by steaming. Trim off the woody ends and stand the asparagus upright inside a clean food tin (with label removed). Stand the tin inside a saucepan of boiling water, the water level being lower than the tin, and cover. Reduce the heat to a simmer and leave the asparagus to steam-cook for around 10–15 minutes. Use tongs or oven gloves to remove the tin and carefully empty the contents onto a plate. Serve with a knob of good-quality margarine or butter, or a drizzle of olive oil and a squeeze of lemon juice. Allow 4 or 5 asparagus spears per person.

For Dinner

ARTICHOKE HEARTS, BROAD BEANS and SHIITAKE MUSHROOMS

This recipe contains beans, which are high in soluble and insoluble fibre, and artichokes, which are a good source of FOS to promote good digestive health. Shiitake are Japanese mushrooms that have many health-giving properties, including the ability to stimulate the immune system. They are available from most large stores, fresh or dried. If dried, rinse and soak for 40 minutes and remove the stems before cooking.

Ingredients
2 tbsp olive oil
2 tbsp ground cumin
1 bay leaf
1 tsp turmeric
250 g (8 oz) shiitake mushrooms, halved
450 g (1 lb) broad beans, de-podded
450 g (1 lb) artichoke hearts, cooked
100 ml (4 fl oz) water
2 tbsp lemon juice
1 small bunch parsley, finely chopped
salt and pepper to taste

Method
Heat the oil gently in a large pan. Add the spices, then the mushrooms. Sauté for a few minutes, then add the broad beans, artichokes and water. Heat through, simmer until the beans are tender, then add the lemon juice and the parsley. Season and serve. Serves four.

SPICY LENTIL CROQUETTES

Lentils are rich in fibre for a healthy digestive system and a source of good-quality vegetable protein. Split red lentils do not need presoaking and so are easy to use. These tasty croquettes can be served hot with cooked vegetables for a main meal, or cold with mixed salad. Always choose organic free-range eggs.

Ingredients
2 sticks of celery, peeled and finely chopped
1 onion, peeled and finely chopped
1 clove garlic, crushed
225 g (8 oz) split red lentils
600 ml (1 pint) water
2 tsp garam masala
1 medium egg
salt and pepper
2 tbsp wholemeal flour
1 tsp turmeric
1 tsp paprika, and 4 tbsp olive oil

Method
Place the celery, onions, garlic, lentils, water and garam masala in a large saucepan. Bring to the boil while stirring. Simmer for 30 minutes, stirring frequently, until the liquid is absorbed and the lentils are tender. Remove from heat and allow to cool for 23 minutes. Add the egg and seasoning and beat in well. Spread the mixture on a plate and allow to cool, then refrigerate for 30–40 minutes. With flour-covered hands, mould the mixture into eight circles. Mix the flour with the turmeric and paprika and use to coat the croquettes. Refrigerate for a further 30–40 minutes. Fry over a moderate heat, turning occasionally, until golden. Makes eight – enough to serve four people.

BRAISED CHICORY
Chicory (endive) is the richest of all natural sources of FOS and makes a piquant accompaniment to any meal. This method of cooking ensures that the chicory is tender.

Ingredients
60 g (2 oz) margarine (or butter)
1 tbsp olive oil
700 g (1½lb) chicory, trimmed and washed
3 tbsp water
1 tsp lemon juice or wine vinegar
½ tsp salt
¼ tsp black pepper

Method
Preheat the oven to 150° C/300° F/Gas 2. Rub half the margarine over the

bottom of a shallow flameproof casserole large enough to hold all the chicory in one layer and arrange the chicory heads in the casserole. Cut the remaining margarine into small pieces and dot them over the chicory. Sprinkle the olive oil over the top. Add the water, lemon juice or vinegar and $\frac{1}{4}$ tsp salt. Place the casserole over a moderate heat and bring the liquid to the boil. Cover the chicory with aluminium foil, put the lid on the casserole and place it in the oven. Braise for $1\frac{1}{4}$ hours, or until the chicory is tender when pierced with a knife. Season the vegetables with the remaining salt and the pepper and serve with any fish, meat or vegetable dish. Serves four.

COUNTRY CASSEROLE

This recipe contains buckwheat, a high-fibre cereal that is never served refined. It has been a staple food in Russia for centuries and is now growing in popularity throughout the world. The red split lentils featured in the recipe can be added straight from the packet – they do not need soaking.

Ingredients
450 ml ($\frac{3}{4}$ pt) water
salt and freshly ground black pepper
150 g (5 oz) buckwheat
2 tbsp vegetable oil
1 red or green pepper, cored, seeded and cut into strips
1 onion, skinned and finely chopped
350 g (12 oz) courgettes, trimmed and sliced
175 g (6 oz) mushrooms, sliced
225 g (8 oz) red split lentils
3 bay leaves
2 tbsp lemon juice
1 garlic clove, skinned and crushed
2 rosemary sprigs
1 tsp cumin seeds
600 ml (1 pt) vegetable stock (or dissolved stock cube in water)
25 g (1 oz) low-fat margarine
chopped fresh parsley, to garnish

Method
Place the water in a saucepan and bring to the boil. Add a pinch of salt, then sprinkle in the buckwheat and return to the boil. Boil rapidly for 1 minute. Reduce the heat, cover and cook gently for 12 minutes or until the water has been absorbed. Do not stir. Transfer to a greased covered dish. Heat the oil in

a flameproof casserole and fry the pepper and onion for 5 minutes. Add the courgettes and mushrooms and fry for a further 5 minutes. Stir in the lentils, lemon juice, garlic, herbs and stock. Add to the casserole and stir well. Simmer for about 45 minutes until the lentils are cooked, stirring occasionally. Add the margarine, adjust the seasoning and sprinkle with parsley. Serve hot with crusty bread or brown rice. Serves four.

Cakes and Desserts

ALMOND MACAROONS

Ingredients
2 egg whites
25 g (1 oz) FOS powder
75 g (3 oz) ground almonds
1 tsp almond essence

Method
Preheat the oven to 120° C/300° F/Gas 2. Whisk the egg whites until they form peaks, and then fold in the FOS powder and almonds with a metal spoon. Add the almond essence and stir. Drop 1 tsp each of the mixture onto a well-oiled baking tray, taking care to leave room for the macaroons to spread out during cooking. Bake for 20 minutes. When cooked, lift off from tray using a palette knife.

BANANA CAKE
This delicious cake includes a multiple helping of FOS, because it is not only in the powder but in the banana as well. Ideally, choose organic free-range eggs, which are tastier and safer than barn eggs. You can use gluten-free flour if you prefer.

Ingredients
1 ripe banana
50 g (2 oz) margarine (or soft butter)
2 medium eggs
50 g (2 oz) FOS powder
150 g (5 oz) flour
1 tsp baking powder

Method

Preheat the oven to 150° C/300° F/Gas 2. Place the banana, margarine (or butter), eggs and FOS powder in a food processor and blend. Transfer to a large bowl. Add the flour and baking powder and beat well. Put into a small lined cake tin (16 cm x 10 cm). Place in the oven and bake for 40 minutes or until a clean knife inserted into the cake comes out clean. Remove from oven and leave to stand for 10 minutes, then turn out onto a wire cooling rack and allow to cool.

CARROT CAKE

This recipe can aid the digestive system in two ways. It contains FOS, to feed the friendly bacteria, and cinnamon, with its proven anti-pathogenic properties. Always choose organic free-range eggs. You can use gluten-free flour if you wish.

Ingredients

2 medium eggs (beaten)
100 g (4 oz) margarine (or soft butter)
175 g (6 oz) finely grated carrots
225 g (8 oz) flour
1 tsp baking powder
50 g (2 oz) FOS powder
1 tsp cinnamon

Method

Preheat the oven to 150° C/300° F/Gas 2. Mix the eggs and margarine (or butter) together, fold in the grated carrot, sift and then add the flour, FOS powder and baking powder to the mixture, along with the cinnamon. Place in a well-oiled tin (22 cm x 11 cm). Bake for 1 hour or until a clean knife inserted into the cake comes out clean. Remove from oven and leave to stand for 10 minutes, then turn out onto a wire cooling rack and allow to cool.

CARROT AND COCONUT CAKE

The mixed spice and coconut in this cake promote a healthy digestive system, as does the FOS powder. Make sure the egg is organic and free range.

Ingredients

175 g (6 oz) finely grated carrot
50 g (2 oz) desiccated coconut

1 tbsp olive oil
1 tsp mixed spice
175 ml (6 fl oz) warm water
150 g (5 oz) brown rice flour
2 tsp baking powder
1 egg
50 g (2 oz) FOS powder

Method
Preheat the oven to 200° C/400° F/Gas 6. Blend all the ingredients in a food processor. Pour into a small well-oiled cake tin. Bake for 40 minutes or until a clean knife inserted in the cake comes out clean. Remove from oven and leave to stand for 10 minutes, then turn out onto a wire cooling rack and allow to cool.

COCONUT PYRAMIDS
Both the FOS powder and the coconut promote good digestive health.

Ingredients
whites of 2 medium eggs
50 g (2 oz) FOS powder
175 g (6 oz) desiccated coconut

Method
Preheat the oven to 150° C/300° F/Gas 2. Whisk the egg whites until stiff. Fold in the FOS powder and the coconut. On a well-oiled baking tray, shape the mixture into pyramids. Bake for 15 minutes.

CRUMBLE TOPPING
This delicious dish is milk-, sugar- and gluten-free and can be used as a topping for any fruits that you like or that are in season.

Ingredients
75 g (3 oz) brown rice flour
75 g (3 oz) margarine (or butter)
75 g (3 oz) ground almonds
50 g (2oz) FOS powder
seasonal fruits of choice

Method
Preheat the oven to 200° C/400° F/Gas 6. Rub together the flour and margarine (or butter) until it resembles fine crumbs. Add the almonds and FOS powder. Place the seasonal fruits in an ovenproof dish, sprinkle over the crumb mixture and bake for 20 minutes. Serves four.

DRIED FRUIT COMPOTE
A compote is any dish of fruit preserved or cooked in syrup. Here, the syrup comes from the natural fruit sugar in the orange juice and dried fruit.

Ingredients
50 g (2 oz) dried apple rings
50 g (2 oz) dried apricots
50 g (2 oz) dried figs
300 ml (½pt) unsweetened orange juice
300 ml (½ pt) water
25 g (1 oz) hazelnuts

Method
Cut the dried apples, apricots and figs into chunky pieces and place in a bowl. Mix together the unsweetened orange juice and water and pour over the fruit in the bowl. Cover and leave to soak in the fridge overnight. When ready to serve, spread the hazelnuts out in a grill pan and toast under a low to moderate heat, shaking the pan frequently until the hazelnuts are browned evenly on all sides. Tip the hazelnuts into a clean tea-towel and rub them while they are still hot to remove the skins. Chop the hazelnuts roughly using an automatic chopper or large cook's knife. Sprinkle over the compote just before serving. Serves six.

FLAPJACKS
This tasty treat is packed with healthy ingredients including oats, sunflower seeds, FOS powder and cinnamon.

Ingredients
50 g (2 oz) margarine (or butter)
100 g (4 oz) porridge oats
25 g (1 oz) sunflower seeds
50 g (2 oz) FOS powder
½ tsp cinnamon

Method
Preheat the oven to 190° C/375° F/Gas 5. Melt the margarine (or butter) in a small saucepan, add the oats, seeds, FOS powder and cinnamon and stir. Place the mixture in a small tin tray. Bake for 30 minutes. Allow to cool and cut into portions, as required.

LEMON MERINGUE PIE
This recipe contains FOS for healthy digestion. Choose organic free-range eggs – and gluten-free flour, if you wish.

Ingredients
Pastry case:
100 g (4 oz) flour
50 g (2 oz) firm margarine (or cold chopped butter)
1 tbsp water
Lemon sauce:
4 tbsp cornflour
75 g (3 oz) FOS powder
25 g (1 oz) margarine (or butter)
3 lemons
Meringue:
4 eggs (separated)
50 g (2 oz) FOS powder

Method
Preheat the oven to 200° C/400° F/Gas 6. In a food processor add flour, 50 g (2 oz) margarine (or butter) and 1 tbsp water and mix until balled. Roll out gently using extra flour. Press into an oiled flan dish. Prick the pastry to prevent rising. Bake blind for 10 minutes. (To bake blind, place a round of greaseproof paper over the pastry and cover with dried haricot beans.) Meanwhile, heat 450 ml (15 fl oz) water with cornflour and FOS powder until thick, stirring continuously. Add the rind and juice of the lemons. When cold, add egg yolks and mix. Remove greaseproof paper and beans. Place the lemon sauce in the pastry case before it sets. Reduce the oven to 150° C/300° F/Gas 2. Beat the 4 egg whites until peaks form, fold in the FOS powder and place onto the pie. Place in the oven for 20 minutes. When cool, keep in the fridge and use within one day.

STUFFED BAKED APPLES

This dish not only includes FOS for a healthy digestive tract, but also cinnamon and mixed spices, which have proven anti-pathogenic properties. FOS powder makes an ideal caster sugar substitute because it is sweet but calorie-free!

Ingredients
4 apples
50 g (2 oz) mixed fruit
25 g (1 oz) FOS powder
1 tsp mixed spice
150 ml (5 fl oz) boiling water
pinch of cinnamon

Method
Preheat the oven to 180° C/350° F/Gas 4. Core the apples and score a line around the outside. Stuff with the dried fruit mixture, FOS powder and cinnamon. Put into an ovenproof dish and surround them with the water. Sprinkle a little more FOS powder over the tops of the apples and bake for 25–30 minutes.

Cocktails

STRAWBERRY ENERGIZER

A great non-alcoholic aperitif, this fruit cocktail is rich in B vitamins to help you extract maximum energy from your food as well as probiotic bacteria to promote digestive health.

Ingredients
6 strawberries, cored and chopped
68 grapes, seedless
2 plums, stoned and chopped
crushed ice
225 ml (8 fl oz) soya milk
1 or 2 bottles of live yoghurt drink

Method
Place all the ingredients in a food processor and blend. Transfer to a suitable container and refrigerate. Serve chilled in two tall glasses.

FRUIT SHAKER

Full of vitamins, this drink makes a great pick-me-up after a hard day. It also contains fibre and cranberry juice for good digestive health.

Ingredients
a handful of chopped blackcurrants, strawberries and raspberries
crushed ice
225 ml (8 fl oz) grape juice
225 ml (8 fl oz) cranberry juice

Method
Place all the ingredients in a food processor and blend. Transfer to a suitable container and refrigerate. Serve chilled in two tall glasses.

Chapter Ten

Food Poisoning and How to Avoid It

The Greek physician Hippocrates, writing in 400 BC said, 'A bad digestion is the root of all evil.' In many cases, the cycle of symptoms that are the hallmark of IBS were first triggered by gastrointestinal infection, through contaminated food.

Many sufferers find their symptoms are worse when they travel abroad – especially when they eat an unfamiliar cuisine. In part, this may be because of holiday stress, or that meals are richer or spicier than they are used to. However, you are also at greater risk of food poisoning when travelling abroad, on holiday, on business or when visiting relatives. Even in parts of the world normally regarded as safe, you will be coming into contact with unfamiliar organisms to which you have no natural immunity.

Medium-risk countries include Portugal, Spain and Turkey. High-risk destinations include Africa, Asia, Latin America and the Middle East.

The Risks

In most cases, gastrointestinal symptoms are mild enough to be dismissed as overindulgence in food or drink. However, food poisoning is potentially very serious – sometimes even fatal. Some groups are at greater risk than others, such as infants, the elderly, pregnant women, and those whose immune system is compromised by disease (HIV/AIDS sufferers, for example) or medication (organ transplant recipients).

As a group, IBS sufferers are not especially prone to food poisoning. But the effects can be more severe and longer lasting in IBS patients than in many non-sufferers. In addition, the incidence of food poisoning is on the increase, at home and abroad. So it makes sense to guard against it. The main ways to protect yourself from food poisoning are: first, strengthen your body's natural defences, and second, try to avoid contamination.

Self-defence

The best self-defence is to ensure your gut is well stocked with friendly bacteria, as explained in Chapter Three. Many experts recommend taking probiotics for at least five days before your holiday starts, and to continue taking them throughout your holiday. This can reduce the risk of digestive upset by up to 30 per cent.

You can pack probiotics as tablets, capsules or sachets, which are available from health food shops and by mail order or via the Internet. Many of these products contain both the beneficial bacteria and the prebiotics they need to thrive. If using sachets, you can mix the powder with pure bottled water or bottled fruit juice, or add them to a hot beverage, or sprinkle over food – but always allow the food or drink to cool first, or you will kill off the bacteria. You may be able to obtain probiotic yoghurt or yoghurt drinks while on holiday, but make sure they come from a trustworthy source.

Acid Barrier
The body's first line of defence is the hydrochloric acid produced in the stomach. Most potentially harmful bacteria that enter the digestive tract in contaminated food are killed by stomach acid. (Probiotic bacteria are resistant to gastric juices, and some have been specially developed to pass through the stomach largely unscathed.)

However, if you use antacid remedies you will breach this vital barrier. Most over-the-counter remedies for excess acid take the form of tablets, chews, powders or liquids containing alkaline chemicals such as hydrogen carbonate, magnesium sulphate and/or aluminium hydroxide. These chemicals neutralize acid to calm an upset stomach. But this also allows food-poisoning germs to pass straight through to the bowel, where they take root, multiply, enter body cells and/or produce toxins.

It is no coincidence that those who over-indulge in alcohol and rich food while on holiday and then take antacids to ease their dyspepsia are most likely to fall prey to 'holiday tummy'. They have, in effect, left themselves wide open to food poisoning. So avoid using antacids while on holiday, or in any other situation where there is a strong risk of coming into contact with food poisoning organisms (see below). Obviously, this also means reducing the need for antacids by, for example, limiting your alcohol consumption and avoiding rich, highly spiced or unfamiliar foods.

The Silent Menace
There are many forms of food poisoning organism. Travellers are often warned about the more serious forms and take precautions. But most pathogens do not get a mention. In part, this is because the inhabitants of the countries you may be visiting are immune to their own local germs and so are unaffected. As only visitors who lack this immunity fall prey to infection, food poisoning cases may go unreported. This can lead to complacency and lack of care when cooks and waiters are preparing food

and drink, increasing the risk of contamination.

Many travellers give little thought to their choice of food venue, perhaps assuming that the same hygiene laws apply abroad as at home. Sadly, this is not always so. Some food poisoning organisms produce toxins that cause sickness only an hour or so after infection. More often, symptoms appear 12-48 hours later. In most cases, symptoms are relatively mild and pass after a few days. Occasionally, the condition is more serious.

Treating Food Poisoning

With mild food poisoning, the best approach is to take plenty of rest and drink lots of fluids. Rehydration powders (electrolyte mixture) are available from pharmacies, which replace the vital salts lost through vomiting and diarrhoea and so aid recovery. Some travellers carry such powders, usually containing salts and glucose, just in case.

You can make your own rehydration drink using 250 ml (9 fl oz) of fruit juice or bottled water mixed with one teaspoon of sugar and a generous pinch of salt.

Try to avoid using anti-diarrhoea drugs unless really necessary (for example, if you have a plane to catch) as they prevent the pathogens being flushed out of the body. In the case of serious illness, especially if accompanied by fever and the passage of blood and/or mucus, seek immediate medical help.

Know Your Enemy

Listed below are some of the commonest food poisoning organisms.

- *Campylobacter jejuni* causes abdominal cramps and diarrhoea. It is mainly spread by poor hygiene practices during food preparation, such as when handling and cooking poultry. In many countries, including the United States, it is now the most common cause of food poisoning. *Campylobacter* can also cause Reiter syndrome, a form of arthritis, and Guillain-Barré syndrome, which can lead to paralysis.
- *Clostridium botulinum* causes a mercifully rare form of poisoning called botulism. This potentially fatal condition is associated mainly with food consumed from old and damaged cans and poorly bottled preserves, such as jam. It is the toxin the bacterium produces that is deadly, rather than the organism itself. Symptoms of botulism include nausea, vomiting, double vision and swallowing problems.

- *Clostridium perfringens* is resistant to high temperatures and so can survive in undercooked stews and pies, especially if incorrectly stored. Symptoms include nausea, vomiting, diarrhoea and abdominal cramps.
- *Entamoeba histolytica* is a single-celled parasite, a type of amoeba, spread by contaminated water, or the food washed in it. The parasite causes amoebic dysentery, with symptoms including abdominal cramps, fever, and the passage of watery diarrhoea and sometimes blood and mucus.
- *Escherichia coli* 0157 is associated mainly with raw meat that is contaminated during the slaughtering process. E. coli is easily destroyed by cooking. Most outbreaks result from cross-contamination, when fresh or cooked food comes into contact with raw meat or the work surfaces and utensils used in its preparation. Symptoms include nausea, diarrhoea, abdominal cramps, headache, fever and malaise.
- *Listeria monocytogenes* infection (listeriosis) is relatively rare and causes listeriosis – flu-like symptoms, including slight fever general aching, and sometimes diarrhoea. It is associated mainly with dairy products, cook-chill meals and salads. Listeriosis is usually mild. More severe symptoms include diarrhoea and abdominal cramps. It poses a serious risk to infants, elderly people and the seriously ill. Pregnant women are especially vulnerable, as listeria infection can cause miscarriage.
- *Salmonella enteriditis* is the most common of all the organisms responsible for salmonella poisoning (salmonellosis), causing abdominal cramps and nausea, diarrhoea, shivering and fever. It is mainly spread in contaminated eggs and poultry. A related food poisoning bacterium, *Salmonella typhimurium*, is associated with mice infestation.
- *Shigella sonnei* (and other members of the *Shigella* group) causes bacterial dysentery. Like amoebic dysentery, this is potentially a very serious condition. Symptoms include abdominal pain, fever, passage of watery diarrhoea and sometimes blood and mucus.
- *Staphylococcus aureus* is a toxin-forming organism commonly found on the skin and can cause septic abscesses. Most outbreaks are traced to poor food handling, especially by people with uncovered wounds and sores.
- Astravirus, hepatitis A, norovirus, Norwalk virus and rotavirus are viral organisms mainly found in food that has been washed in contaminated water or been in contact with an infected person. Symptoms include vomiting, diarrhoea, headache, abdominal cramps, fever and, in

severe cases, shock and collapse. Outbreaks are most common where holidaymakers are in close proximity for long periods, such as in holiday camps and on cruise ships.

Outbreaks of the most deadly food poisoning diseases, such as cholera (*Vibrio cholerae*) and typhoid *(Salmonella typhi)*, tend to be confined to poorer regions of the world, where sanitation is primitive, especially during times of conflict and disaster. You are advised to get vaccinated before travelling in areas where diseases such as cholera and typhoid are endemic (in some countries, a vaccination certificate is a condition of entry). It is also possible to be vaccinated against viral hepatitis A.

What Are the Main Risks?

Most food poisoning occurs because of cross-contamination, either because of poor hygiene (for example, not washing hands after visiting the lavatory), or when raw meat, fish and eggs come into contact with cooked meats, salads and pre-prepared meals. In the United Kingdom, you are most at risk when eating out, in a restaurant or café, and at social events such as barbecues or catered events such as conferences or wedding receptions.

People take more care when preparing meals in their own kitchens, washing their hands thoroughly and keeping utensils and work surfaces scrupulously clean. But mistakes can occur through lack of concentration, especially when under time pressure, or through poor storage and preparation. Common-sense measures can limit the risks.

Food Safety in the Home
Good hygiene is obviously the first priority. It is not enough just to wash your hands before starting to prepare food. Many raw foods are contaminated. It is easy to spread germs to kitchen utensils, plates, cutlery and then to the food after it has been cooked before serving. So wash your hands frequently when preparing food, especially after handling raw meat, fish and eggs. Choose plastic (polypropylene) chopping boards in preference to wooden ones, which can harbour germs, and disinfect them regularly.

Ensure that chopping boards, plates and utensils used for preparing raw meat and fish are not also used for cooked food and fresh vegetables. Place the board, knives and other utensils in hot soapy water in the sink as soon as you have finished with them.

Wash dishes, plates, cutlery and other utensils in hot water (wear rubber gloves), using a good-quality washing-up liquid, and then rinse under hot running water before placing on a draining board. If left for an hour or so, the dishes may be dry enough to put away. Otherwise, dry with paper kitchen towel or a freshly laundered tea towel (replaced daily).

Storage
Correct storage is vitally important. In warm conditions (5–60° C/40–140° F) harmful bacteria multiply rapidly to dangerous levels. A common food poisoning bacterium such as *E. coli 0157* can double every 20 minutes. This means that a single *E. coli* can become a colony of a million in just seven hours. So it is important to reduce the time that raw food remains within this temperature range. Even rice and cereals pose a threat. If not stored correctly, these foods can harbour the bacterium *Bacillus cereus*, which multiplies rapidly in rice and pasta dishes.

Bacterial cell growth slows down or stops altogether in cold or icy conditions, so make sure your refrigerator and freezer are at the correct temperature (fridge below 4° C/39° F and the freezer at −18° C/−1° F or below). If you are in any doubt about the temperature, buy a special fridge/freezer thermometer and check.

Carry chilled and frozen food home in an insulated cooler bag or box and refrigerate soon after purchase. Make sure frozen food is defrosted thoroughly before cooking, and never re-freeze food that has been defrosted unless it has been cooked right through. Most bacteria are destroyed by temperatures over 75° C/17° F. Ensure that reheated food is piping hot before serving, and never reheat food more than once. Cooked food intended for storage should be taken out of the oven, covered, and left to cool before refrigerating. (If the kitchen is warm, consider transferring to a cooler room.)

Store raw meat and fish in sealed plastic bags or containers in the fridge, and take care not to let blood or other fluid drip onto foods. Chicken and pork are among the worst offenders, but all raw meat and fish is a potential source of contamination.

'Use by' Dates
Food that can spoil and become unsafe over time must, by law, have a 'use by' date printed on the packaging. This includes all meat, fish and eggs, and some dairy products, fresh or cooked foods, and prepared salads. As a general rule, any food kept in a store's refrigerator or freezer cabinet, or stored on ice (in the case of fish and shellfish), has a limited storage life and should be consumed on or before the date specified. Never eat food that has exceeded its 'use by' date, even if it looks, smells and tastes acceptable, as harmful bacteria may have built up to dangerous levels.

Foods that deteriorate quickly often carry a 'display by' date as well. This is a guide to food retailers and helps ensure that only the highest quality food is on sale. 'Use by' should not be confused with a 'best before' date. Dried, packet or canned foods generally have a long shelf-life but the quality may deteriorate over time, losing flavour or becoming stale. The 'best before' date indicates how long a food remains good quality. After this date the food may still be safe to eat, provided the packaging is intact and the food appears and smells wholesome.

Most canned foods will last from one to three years. Once opened, however, canned food should be treated as highly perishable and eaten immediately, or transferred to a suitable container and refrigerated. Consume within 48 hours.

Seafood Risks
Seafood, both fish and shellfish, is highly nutritious, packed with protein, fatty acids (omega-3) and minerals such as iodine and zinc that a healthy body needs, and so are important components of a balanced diet. Well-known brands of pre-prepared seafood are usually perfectly safe. However, fresh seafood can pose a risk unless obtained from a reputable source and correctly stored and cooked. Many forms of shellfish, such as oysters and mussels, are filter feeders and accumulate pathogenic microbes. Fish, too, can harbour harmful organisms in large numbers unless kept cold. You can avoid most risks by taking simple precautions.

Buying Shellfish
Always obtain fresh shellfish from a reputable source, such as a well-known store or fishmonger. These shellfish come from coastal waters that must meet strict national and international standards on cleanliness. Avoid shellfish that comes from an unknown supplier, especially if being offered suspiciously cheap.

Make sure the shells of oysters and mussels you buy are tightly closed – or close when you touch them – as this shows they are alive. Prawns should have translucent, unbroken shells. Cook all shellfish thoroughly – mussels, for example, should be steamed for at least six minutes.

Buying Fish
Whole fish on sale in shops, stores and stalls should be displayed on a bed of ice. If cut into portions such as fillets and steaks, fish should be kept on trays, paper or plastic film either on ice or in a refrigerated cabinet. Good-quality fish has a fresh, almost 'sweet' smell, with moist, shiny scales, bright pink or red gills and clear bulging eyes. Fish portions should have firm, moist, non-slimy flesh.

Whole fish should be refrigerated – not frozen – as soon as possible and cleaned and cooked within 24 hours of purchase. Fish portions can be stored in the freezer for a few days, but then defrosted thoroughly and cooked right through. Do not re-freeze.

Raw Fish Dishes
Japanese sushi and sashimi dishes feature raw fish, which in rare cases can carry parasites, such as a roundworm called anisakis. Good-quality Japanese restaurants employ skilled sushi chefs who know how to identify and remove fish parasites. But be wary of eating sushi except in well-established venues. If you are tempted to prepare sushi yourself, obtain your fish from reputable stores (employing experienced fishmongers) and say what you want the fish for, so they can ensure that it is safe.

Eggs and Poultry
Take care when handling eggs and poultry. Meat and shells may be contaminated with Salmonella bacteria, among other pathogens. When buying eggs, check that the shells are undamaged and unsoiled. Opt for organic free-range eggs, rather than 'farm' or 'barn' eggs, which come from battery farms and so are highly likely to be contaminated.

Eggs need not be kept refrigerated, but should be stored in their carton in a cool place, such as a larder, and eaten within two weeks of purchase. To test for freshness submerge eggs in water – if they sink they are fresh. Stale eggs generate gas, which makes them float. Wipe the shells before you crack them open and then dispose of the shells and wash your hands immediately.

To ensure that eggs are thoroughly cooked, check that all the 'white' is indeed white and not translucent, and that the yolk has started to set. As a guide, cook boiled eggs for at least 8 minutes, poached for at least 6 minutes and scrambled for at least 3 minutes. Avoid recipes that feature raw egg, such as cheesecake, ice cream, mayonnaise, mousse, sorbet and soufflé. Shop brands from reputable sources are safe as commercial food producers use pasteurized eggs, which are sterile.

Defrost poultry thoroughly and make sure it is cooked right through before serving. *Salmonella* is killed by high temperatures only, so cool, undercooked parts inside a chicken or turkey can harbour germs that multiply rapidly. To test that the meat is fully cooked, push a clean skewer deep into the body of the bird. The juices that flow out should be clear. Any blood or pink coloration shows that the meat is undercooked.

Cheese
Some types of cheese carry increased risk, particularly from *Listeria*. Most at risk are the very young, the elderly, pregnant women, and those with a

compromised immune system. The main risk comes from poor handling, so contamination is most likely to be found on the surface, especially the rind.

Cheeses to be wary of include soft types, such as Brie, and blue-veined kinds, such as Stilton. To be safe, buy from reputable outlets only. Hard cheeses, such as Cheddar, Cheshire, Parmesan and Red Leicester, have higher acidity levels, which helps control pathogen levels, and so are regarded as safe. Cheese made from unpasteurized milk is not thought to pose any additional risk.

Barbecues

It takes skill to cook foods thoroughly on a barbecue. The fierce heat of a charcoal fire can seal the surface of foods such as burgers, sausages and chops, leaving the inside underdone. Check that food is cooked right through before serving (especially chicken wings and drumsticks, which take longer to cook through). Avoid foods that are blackened on one side and raw on the other, or pink in the centre. To be safe, pre-cook food in an oven and finish off on the barbecue for a charcoal-grilled flavour. Keep uncooked items such as salads, dips and mayonnaise in the fridge until ready to serve and then place on ice or in a coolbox.

Eating Away from Home

Be wary of buffet meals if the food is left uncovered at room temperature for long periods. If there is a choice, opt for a hot meal rather than cold food. Otherwise, limit yourself to a few 'safe' choices. Don't be tempted to sample several different dishes just to see what they are like: this increases the risk that a food you choose is contaminated.

Holiday Safety

All holidaymakers are at risk when travelling abroad. But for reasons that are unclear, UK holidaymakers seem to be far more vulnerable to food poisoning than other European tourists. Overindulgence in food and alcohol and use of antacids (see above) may be factors. Perhaps Britons more readily succumb to the holiday mood and throw caution to the winds. However, at the risk of curbing your holiday spirit, bear in mind that a gastrointestinal upset will not only blight your holiday, but may also damage your long-term health and wellbeing.

Dine Out with Care

Steer clear of pavement food vendors and avoid restaurants and cafés where flies congregate or that allow refuse to pile up (a magnet for rats and cockroaches). Good restaurants let you inspect the kitchens beforehand; be wary of any that refuse your request.

Unless you have total confidence in the hygiene standards of the restaurant or hotel you visit, choose hot foods in preference to cold meals such as salads, and insist that the meal is served piping hot to the table. Avoid raw fish and shellfish (such as sushi and oysters), and food left uncovered. Choose fruits you can peel yourself.

Don't have ice in drinks, and opt for boiled, bottled, canned or carton drinks, which should be served with the seal intact (bottled fruit juices may be watered down). Otherwise choose carbonated (fizzy) drinks and sparkling bottled water. Hot drinks such as coffee and tea are usually safe, but avoid adding cow's, sheep's or goat's milk unless pasteurized. This also applies to products made from milk, such as cream, cheese and ice cream. If you buy milk, always boil it before drinking.

Tap water smelling strongly of chlorine is probably safe, but may taste unpleasant. Therefore for general use, for example drinks, washing fruit and cleaning your teeth, buy bottled water (again, check that the seal is intact) or boil the water for at least five minutes.

Another approach is to use a water purifier. Some types have a pump action and incorporate an iodine resin and charcoal filter. Or you can sterilize water with tincture of iodine (available from pharmacists) or chemical sterilization tablets, which usually also contain iodine. Leave for 30 minutes before using. Whatever form of purification you choose, be sure that it is guaranteed to remove or kill all disease organisms – bacteria, viruses and parasites. Bear in mind that *Entamoeba histolyca* is resistant to chlorine types.

Safe Bathing

Take care, too, when bathing. A swimming pool is safe if it smells of chlorine, but otherwise should be avoided. Many waterways are contaminated with raw sewage and industrial waste. Before you swim in the sea, lake or river, check with a reliable source, such as your hotel or the local tourist information office, to make sure that it is safe.

Chapter Eleven

Stress and Other Factors

There are many aspects of your lifestyle that may be contributing to your symptoms, in addition to diet. To manage your condition effectively, you should give some thought to all areas of your life. The lifestyle factors that can make the biggest difference to IBS sufferers are stress levels, exercise, alcohol intake and smoking.

Of these, managing your stress levels is the first one to tackle. Reducing stress is important to health for many reasons, not just to help alleviate IBS. Chronic (long-term) stress is associated with high blood pressure, excess smoking and drinking, depression, anxiety, high blood cholesterol, heart disease and stroke, among other problems.

This should persuade you to deal with the causes of stress (or 'stressors') in your life. It may mean having to make difficult decisions in order to solve the underlying issue(s). But it is better to tackle them now, rather than wait till your health is seriously affected and the stressors have still not gone away. Once you start to manage stress you may find it easier to tackle other problem areas such as drinking, comfort eating and smoking, all of which tend to increase in direct proportion to the tension you feel.

The Need to De-stress

As part of your stress management regime you will need to:

- understand how stress can both trigger and exacerbate your IBS symptoms.
- recognize stressors in your life and eliminate them, or try to accept them and learn how to cope with them better.
- include periods of relaxation in your day, for example, using breathing and relaxation techniques, guides and tapes.

The Stress Response

Before looking at how to manage stress, it helps to understand exactly what stress is. To be 'stressed' means to be put under pressure. Any object that has to cope with a force that pushes it to the limit is under stress. Your body is no exception.

The body's reaction to stress is the 'fight or flight' response, designed to get your body working at maximum to cope with a physical threat. In the right circumstances, this response is a life-saver. It will galvanize you into reacting to danger by, for example, running away from a vicious dog, avoiding a speeding car, leaping from a burning building or fighting off an attacker.

In an emergency, the sympathetic nervous system is triggered and acts on internal organs directly, via nerve pathways, and indirectly, by triggering the release of the stress hormones adrenalin and noradrenalin.

These hormones travel round the bloodstream and act on the lungs, heart, muscles and blood vessels. As a result, the breath quickens, so you take in more oxygen, and the heart beats faster, and blood vessels widen to rush the extra oxygen to the muscles.

Stress hormones mobilize the body's reserves of glucose sugar and fats to fuel your exertions. The adrenal glands also release corticosteroid hormones, such as cortisol to suppress the immune system and so preserve vital energy reserves. Once the crisis passes, your body returns to normal.

Positive and Negative Stress

Thrill-seekers actively look for situations that trigger this response because of the 'adrenalin rush' of excitement they feel when pushing themselves to the limit. Some get a buzz clinching a business contract against all the odds, or through risky sports, like motor racing or rock climbing, or with scary fairground rides. This is called positive stress.

But not all stressors are enjoyable, sought after, or resolved by physical action. For example, if you have a heavy workload and a tight deadline, or are preparing for a big occasion such as a wedding, and are struggling to cope, you react as if facing a physical threat. This is negative stress.

In this case the stress response is inappropriate because you don't need to gear up for physical action. In fact, stress makes the situation worse, because you need a clear head in a crisis like this – and that's difficult when your heart is pounding.

When faced with stressors that cannot be resolved easily, you are in a permanent state of stress. Heart and breathing rate keep high, glucose and fats stay in the blood and the immune system remains suppressed. This is why chronic stress causes such varied physical disorders.

Stress and IBS

The digestive tract is controlled by its own set of nerves, called the enteric system, which controls the muscular movements of the GI tract. During times of stress, however, the sympathetic nerve activity in the bowel increases. As a consequence, not only is the bowel hypersensitive to stimuli, caused by fatty or spicy foods, for example, but the bowel itself behaves in an exaggerated fashion to trigger the symptoms of IBS, such as abdominal pain, diarrhoea and constipation.

Stress Management

Stress management is covered in more detail in the companion book to this one, but in essence there are three phases. Phase one: identify the principal stressors in your life, such as emotional or relationship problems, work and financial worries, and health issues involving you or your family. Phase two: deal with them. Even if you cannot resolve these problems, try to reduce the impact they are having.

It is virtually impossible to eliminate or avoid all of life's stressors, however, so phase three is finding a way to relax, especially whenever under greatest pressure. The most effective relaxation techniques include deep meditation, breathing methods and visualization. These usually work best in combination, for example by combining deep breathing with meditation. However, you may have other ways of dealing with stress. All that matters is that the technique works for you.

Facing Facts

Of course stressors, by their very nature, are never easy to deal with. If they were they wouldn't cause stress. You would simply tackle the problem and the stress would go away. However, half the battle is in accepting that there is a problem. For example, people often let relationship problems drag on indefinitely rather than facing up to the underlying issues. But the very act of admitting that the issue must be dealt with, by talking over the problem with a partner, relative or friend involved, for example, can help reduce stress, even before a solution is found. Similarly, discussing a financial problem with your bank, a close friend or the Citizens Advice Bureau, or seeking a meeting with your boss to discuss a work issue can help put your mind at ease.

Relaxation Techniques

One way to relax is to set aside time for yourself, away from the distractions and irritations that others cause, and just spend time on your own doing what you want to do. This could be relaxing in the bath, listening to music, reading a favourite book, taking long walks, playing sport, watching a film, or doing a hobby such as gardening or crafts.

It seems too simple to be effective, but these vital moments of 'me' time often get squeezed out of a hectic schedule filled with commuting, working, cooking and cleaning, child care and looking after relatives. Try to establish a period in the day to devote to yourself, and make it clear to others that this time is sacrosanct. Once you establish a routine, you will find it much easier to keep to it, and others will learn to respect it, too.

Some people cannot truly relax unless they use a formal technique, such as visualization or meditation, often combined with deep breathing. There are audio tapes and CDs that provide aural background atmosphere, such as the sounds of the shoreline, birdsong or whale music.

Another technique is to find a comfortable seated position and focus on a candle, or an ornament, and let your mind clear completely. If any thought enters your head, acknowledge it but do not dwell on it, and simply allow it to pass out again. At the same time, take slow even breaths, drawing the air deep into your abdomen. This technique may take time to master, but you can use it any time you are feeling stressed.

Another technique is visualization. Here, rather than making your mind blank, you fill your mind with a relaxing image. Use any image that works for you, such as a secluded beach you discovered on holiday, a picnic spot in the country, a comfy chair at a grandparent's house, or your own garden. It should be somewhere you always feel relaxed and a place you can visualize so strongly that you almost feel you are there. As you immerse yourself in the image, the sense of relaxation will grow.

Add plenty of detail to your image. Although it is called 'visualization', try to bring all the senses into play, not just sight. Feel the wind on your face, the sensation of sand running through your fingers, the fabric of the chair, or the grass under your feet. Hear the sound of the waves and the gulls, the wind through the trees, an old grandfather clock, or the murmur of insects. Smell the seaweed, the new-mown hay, the mixture of furniture polish and lavender scent, or the heady aroma of garden flowers.

There are other relaxation techniques to try, singly or in combination, until you find one that works for you.

Exercising More

Regular exercise provides many proven health benefits. It can be beneficial in IBS directly, by improving bowel function, and indirectly, by alleviating stress, tension, anxiety and depression and improving your mental outlook in general. All forms of exercise can aid the bowel's peristaltic (squeezing) action, especially if you are drinking plenty of fluids and have increased your fibre intake.

Exercise need not mean joining a gym or sports club, although these are excellent ways to get fit. Aim to increase your activity levels generally, by walking more and using the car and public transport less. Walk to the shops when you can, rather than use the car, and go for a walk during lunch breaks or whenever you have a few minutes to escape from household chores. Take longer walks in the early evenings and at weekends.

Where possible, vary your activities. For example, include a weekly swimming session, or use a bike from time to time, dig the garden or decorate the spare room. It is a good idea to include a few stretches to aid flexibility, and exercises such as abdominal crunches ('sit-ups') that target the abdomen directly.

Exercise can play an important part in stress management. It helps burn up the sugar and fats that stress releases, and it boosts endorphin levels, the 'feel good' chemicals that lift your spirits. If you are planning to give up smoking (see below), it is a good idea to start a regular exercise routine at the same time. It gives you an excuse to avoid the places you associate with smoking, counteracts craving, and helps control your weight.

Limiting Your Alcohol Intake

Once you have started to minimize your stress levels you should be in a better position to tackle other areas that may be contributing to your symptoms, such as your alcohol intake. Much of drinking is simply habit. In the pub, club or restaurant you might order an alcoholic drink almost automatically or accept one when offered.

Similarly at home, you might pour yourself a drink as soon as you walk through the door, or at a certain time each evening, or have one or more with the evening meal. As a result, your alcohol intake grows, almost imperceptibly, week by week, to a level that could contribute to your IBS symptoms.

Of course, there are many health reasons to moderate alcohol consumption. So think of IBS as a warning. Reduce your alcohol intake now to ease your IBS symptoms, and you will also reduce the burden on your liver, cut back on calories, and reduce the risk of other health disorders. Alcohol can be a boon to health, cutting the risk of heart disease and stroke, for example – but only in moderation. In excess, it increases the risk.

If you think your alcohol intake may be too high, make a note in your food diary (see Chapter Two) of each drink you consume each day. As a general guide, most health experts advise no more than two glasses of beer, wine or spirit a day and have to two or three alcohol-free days each week to give your liver a chance to recover.

Diluting wine with soda water, or drinking shandy instead of beer, will make an alcoholic drink go further for the same number of units. In pubs and clubs, alternate alcoholic drinks with colas and fruit juices, or choose low-alcohol beer, and drink water instead of wine with your meals. Once you break the habit you will find you can manage your units more effectively. The rewards will be better sleep patterns, a trimmer figure, extra cash for other things, and – hopefully – an improvement in IBS symptoms.

Giving up Smoking

The dangers of smoking are too well publicized to need repeating here. If you haven't already made up your mind to quit, there is nothing I could say that would persuade you. But if you want to quit, but are not sure how to go about it, here are some tips that other ex-smokers have found helpful. And that includes me.

- Choose a date to give up that you stand a good chance of keeping to. That means not Christmas or New Year, when your social diary is full and temptation is all around, and not at times of stress, such as before exams or when moving house.
- Tell non-smoking friends, relatives and colleagues of your plan and impress on them how important this is to you. Ask them to help you keep to your resolution.
- Avoid smokers. They are your worst enemy at this time. Whatever they may say, secretly they want you to fail, so expect little help from them.
- Change your routine to avoid pubs, clubs and other places where you normally smoke.
- Spend more time in places where smoking is not allowed, such as the homes of non-smoking friends, libraries, theatres, cinemas, swimming pools and health clubs.
- Take more exercise (see above).
- Avoid high-sugar, high-fat snacks as cigarette substitutes and eat more fruit and vegetables and low-fat snacks such as pretzels and rice cakes.
- Avoid alcohol, tea and coffee for the first few weeks, as these make cravings worse. Drink fruit and vegetable juices, herbal teas and plain water instead.
- Finally, keep busy. Take up a hobby, or catch up on jobs you have been putting off.

Chapter Twelve

Diagnosis and Treatment of IBS

Many IBS sufferers find that a combination of dietary and other lifestyle changes can keep their symptoms under control. In addition, there are various over-the-counter remedies available from pharmacies that relieve troublesome IBS symptoms. But seek your pharmacist's advice before using remedies, as some are not suitable for IBS.

You should take care to avoid over-using medication for IBS, as this can have potentially serious side effects over time. For example, excessive use of laxatives can weaken bowel function and make constipation worse. See your doctor if you are taking over-the-counter medication on a regular basis, or if your symptoms are serious enough to affect the quality of your life and/or restrict your freedom, or if you have any of the 'red flag' symptoms listed in Chapter One.

Diagnosing IBS

Your doctor will ask you about your symptoms and when they occur, and may carry out a physical examination. If your doctor is concerned that there may be an underlying condition, such as allergy, coeliac disease or lactose intolerance, he or she may arrange tests (see below).

In most cases, IBS is diagnosed on the basis of your symptoms (and an absence of the symptoms and signs that might indicate a different condition). Indeed, there is no test that can prove IBS. However, if you follow your doctor's advice regarding diet and other lifestyle changes and take any medication prescribed, and your symptoms improve, this will normally be taken as confirmation of IBS.

Treating IBS

Unless your symptoms are very severe, many doctors will prefer that you try to tackle your symptoms through lifestyle changes, such as diet or stress management (see Chapter Eleven) before prescribing medication. In part, this is because there is no single prescription medicine that has proved effective in all cases of IBS. Most medicines given for IBS simply alleviate symptoms.

If the doctor thinks medication is appropriate, he or she can prescribe a drug such as an antispasmodic that is stronger and more effective than those available from a pharmacy. These drugs relax the smooth muscle in the bowel wall and so help prevent the spasms that cause pain, bloating, constipation and/or diarrhoea.

As well as laxatives or anti-diarrhoeals, you may be prescribed mild painkillers, such as paracetamol, or antacids for indigestion. Low doses of tranquillizers or antidepressants can help some patients. These drugs not only ease the psychological symptoms (such as anxiety) that can trigger or accompany IBS symptoms, but may also target nerve chemicals such as serotonin that help control nerve activity in the bowel (as well as the central nervous system), which are thought to be overactive in IBS sufferers.

Tests for Related Conditions

If your condition does not respond to lifestyle changes and medication (but there are no 'red flag' symptoms and signs to suggest a life-threatening condition; see Chapter One), the doctor may want to rule out other conditions that cause similar symptoms, such as food allergy, coeliac disease and lactose intolerance.

Food Allergy Testing

Patients can normally recognize when they are allergic to a food because they will react to it every time they eat it. Normally, they will try to avoid it. But in the case of foods such as nuts, it may be present in food without the sufferer being aware. Food allergy symptoms include swollen lips, tongue or throat, nausea, abdominal pain, diarrhoea, nettle rash (urticaria), coughing, wheezing, runny nose, swollen eyes and palpitations.

Tests for food allergies are widely available. In serious cases, your doctor may arrange to have the test carried out by doctors known as allergists, who are based at specialist hospital units and clinics. More often, however, people make use of private allergy clinics that specialize in testing and treatment. Standard food allergy tests include the skin prick test and the intradermal test.

In the skin prick test, a solution containing a small amount of a suspect food is placed on the skin. A needle is then used to prick the skin through the solution. More than one potential allergen may be tested at the same time on different areas of skin. Intradermal testing differs from the skin prick test in that the test substance is injected directly into the skin, using a hypodermic needle and syringe.

A positive reaction is indicated by an intense itching occurring one or two minutes later. This shows that the immune response has been activated, causing histamine to be released from special mast cells. Fluid leaks out of tiny blood vessels under the skin, forming a raised blister, or weal, surrounded by a wider area of redness and itching. This initial reaction goes away after a few hours, often leaving a slight swelling at the site. A second, milder reaction may occur the next day.

In theory, a positive reaction shows you are allergic to a food, and a negative reaction indicates that you are not (although you may react to it for other reasons unconnected with an allergy). However, tests for food allergens are less reliable than tests for inhaled or skin-contact allergens, as false positives and false negatives are common. Sometimes the skin reacts to a substance that causes no symptoms when eaten, or a known symptom-provoking food may not trigger a skin reaction at all.

Antihistamines, taken for hay fever, for example, can interfere with the test. So you should stop taking antihistamines before an allergy test. Older people sometimes show a weak response to allergy testing, so results are less conclusive in their case.

There is a more accurate form of allergy testing called the radioallergosorbent test (RAST). This measures blood levels of immunoglobulin E, an antibody associated with allergies, which is released in response to an allergen. This test is not as widely available as other forms of allergy testing.

Allergy Treatment
Allergies can be treated by desensitization, also known as allergy immunotherapy or hyposensitization. This involves a regular course of injections containing tiny quantities of the allergen. The amount given each time is slowly increased so that the immune system becomes more tolerant of the substance and less likely to react.

Injections are usually administered weekly at first, steadily reducing to once a month. Allergy treatment does not usually effect a cure, but can reduce symptoms to tolerable levels in some people. It is less effective in people with food allergies than with other types of allergy.

Desensitization can take several months to take effect, so don't expect immediate results. But if you see no real improvement after a year or two, the treatment is probably not working. Desensitization is expensive, so if you plan to have private treatment, ask the clinician in charge to establish a deadline by which you can expect to see a significant improvement in your symptoms.

Caution
There is a slight risk of a life-threatening reaction called anaphylactic shock following exposure to an allergen. This is most often seen in people with nut

allergy, and less commonly in those allergic to shellfish. For this reason, trained medical staff must be on hand during allergy testing and treatment to administer first aid, such as emergency resuscitation and an injection of adrenalin. Shock can be delayed in some cases, so you must stay at the clinic for at least two hours after testing.

Coeliac Disease Testing and Treatment
A doctor may make an initial diagnosis of coeliac disease based on the symptoms, which can include abdominal pain, diarrhoea, vomiting, bloating, fatigue, weight loss and rash. To confirm the diagnosis, patients are referred to a hospital gastroenterology department for special tests such as a biopsy, in which a small piece of intestine is removed and examined for signs of damage. A biopsy is performed during an endoscopic examination, in which a flexible, fibre-optic viewing device is passed down the throat and, via the stomach, into the small intestine. The endoscope is equipped with small remote-controlled cutting tools to remove the tissue.

The biopsy may be repeated several times over a period of weeks to compare the condition of the intestine after the patient has been eating a diet that contains gluten, and after he or she has been eating a gluten-free diet. There will be a marked difference in the condition of the small intestine between the two sets of tests. Blood and urine may be checked for signs of malabsorption problems, such as iron deficiency anaemia.

If coeliac disease is confirmed, the only solution is to avoid all gluten-containing cereals, including wheat, rye, barley and, in some cases, oats. Usually symptoms improve within a week or two of starting this diet. Coeliacs do not usually have to avoid other types of food, so there is little risk of malnutrition. Occasionally, coeliac disease can cause lactose intolerance (see below).

Lactose Intolerance and Treatment
This condition can be diagnosed on the basis of symptoms, such as abdominal pain, diarrhoea, bloating and flatulence, but can only be confirmed by tests, such as the lactose tolerance test, the hydrogen breath test and the stool acidity test.

In the lactose tolerance test, the patient is given a drink containing lactose and a blood sample is then taken at regular periods of 30 minutes to two hours afterwards. The blood is analysed to detect any rise in glucose, which is produced when lactose is broken down in the small intestine. Absence of or reduced glucose in the blood indicates a lack of the enzyme lactase, needed to digest lactose.

In the hydrogen breath test, the patient is again given a drink containing lactose, but this time the breath is analysed using a device that measures the hydrogen level. The test is repeated several times over a couple of hours. The level of hydrogen in the breath indicates the degree of intolerance to lactose.

In the stool acidity test, a sample of faeces is analysed for its pH (acidity/alkalinity) level. Low pH (high acidity) shows that the small intestine is not digesting lactose efficiently.

Management of lactose intolerance mainly involves avoiding dairy products (apart from yoghurt, which is normally well tolerated). Some sufferers take supplements of lactase so that they can consume milk and other dairy products perfectly normally.

Appendix A: E Numbers

This is the current list of additives to be found in foods at the time of writing, or likely to be approved for use in the near future. It includes some substances under discussion but not yet finally approved for use in foodstuffs. More additives are being considered for inclusion all the time. The following entries have been categorized according to their most common use, but some have more than one function, for example, as stabilizers and thickening agents. Entries marked [A] may cause allergy in some people. If you notice a bad reaction after consuming a food or drink containing one of these additives, it is a good idea to mark the E number with an X as a record of products to avoid.

Key

[A]   Possible cause of allergy
[U]   Probable new number

E number: Common name(s)

Colourings

E number	Common name(s)
E100	Curcumin
E101	(i) Riboflavin
	(ii) Riboflavin-5'-phosphate
E102 [A]	Tartrazine, FD&C Yellow 5
E103	Chrysoine Resorcinol
E104 [A]	Quinoline Yellow
E105	Fast Yellow AB
E106	Riboflavin-5-Sodium Phosphate
E107 [A]	Yellow 2G
E110 [A]	Sunset Yellow FCF, Orange Yellow S
E111	Orange GGN
E120 [A]	Cochineal, Carminic acid, Carmines
E121	Orcein, Orchil
E122 [A]	Azorubine, Carmoisine
E123 [A]	Amaranth, FD&C Red 2
E124 [A]	Ponceau 4R, Cochineal Red A, Brilliant Scarlet 4R
E125	Scarlet GN
E126	Ponceau 6R
E127 [A]	Erythrosine, FD&C Red 3
E128 [A]	Red 2G
E129 [A]	Allura Red AC, FD&C Red 40

E131 [A]	Patent Blue V
E132 [A	Indigotine, Indigo carmine
E133 [A]	Brilliant Blue FCF
E140	(i) Chlorophylls
	(ii) Chlorophyllins
E141	(i) Copper complexes of chlorophylls
	(ii) Copper complexes of chlorophyllins
E142 [A]	Green S
E150a	Plain caramel
E150b	Caustic sulphite caramel
E150c	Ammonia caramel
E150d	Sulphite ammonia caramel
E151 [A]	Brilliant Black BN, Black PN
E152 [A]	Black 7984
E153	Vegetable carbon
E154 [A]	Brown FK
E155 [A]	Brown HT
E160a [A]	(i) Mixed carotenes
	(ii) Beta-carotene
	(iii) Gamma-carotene
E160b	Annatto, bixin, norbixin
E160c	Paprika extract,
	capsanthin, capsorubin
E160d	Lycopene
E160e	Beta-apo-8'-carotenal (C 30)
E160f	Ethyl ester of beta-apo-8'-carotenic acid (C 30)
E161a	Flavoxanthin
E161b	Lutein
E161c	Cryptoaxanthin
E161d	Rubixanthin
E161e	Violaxanthin
E161f	Rhodoxanthin
E161g	Canthaxanthin
E162	Beetroot Red, betanin
E163	Anthocyanins
E170	Calcium carbonates
E171	Titanium dioxide
E172	Iron oxides and hydroxides
E173	Aluminium
E174	Silver
E175	Gold
E180	Latolrubine BK

E181	Tannin

Preservatives

E200	Sorbic acid
E202	Potassium sorbate
E203	Calcium sorbate
E210 [A]	Benzoic acid
E211 [A]	Sodium benzoate
E212 [A]	Potassium benzoate
E213 [A]	Calcium benzoate
E214 [A]	Ethyl p-hydroxybenzoate
E215 [A]	Sodium ethyl p-hydroxybenzoate
E216 [A]	Propyl p-hydroxybenzoate
E217 [A]	Sodium propyl p-hydroxybenzoate
E218 [A]	Methyl p-hydroxybenzoate
E219 [A]	Sodium methyl p-hydroxybenzoate
E220 [A]	Sulphur dioxide
E221 [A]	Sodium sulphite
E222 [A]	Sodium hydrogen sulphite
E223 [A]	Sodium metabisulphite
E224 [A]	Potassium metabisulphite
E226 [A]	Calcium sulphite
E227 [A]	Calcium hydrogen sulphite
E228 [A]	Potassium hydrogen sulphite
E230	Biphenyl, diphenyl
E231	Orthophenyl phenol
E232	Sodium orthophenyl phenol
E234	Nisin
E235	Natamycin
E236	Formic acid
E237	Sodium formiate
E238	Calcium formiate
E239	Hexamethylene tetramine
E242	Dimethyl dicarbonate
E249	Potassium nitrite
E250	Sodium nitrite
E251	Sodium nitrate
E252	Potassium nitrate
E260	Acetic acid
E261	Potassium acetate
E262	(i) Sodium acetate
	(ii) Sodium hydrogen acetate (sodium diacetate)

E263	Calcium acetate
E264	Ammonium acetate
E270	Lactic acid
E280	Propionic acid
E281	Sodium propionate
E282 [A]	Calcium propionate
E283	Potassium propionate
E284	Boric acid
E285	Sodium tetraborate (borax)
	Acidity Regulators
E290	Carbon dioxide
E296	Malic acid
E297	Fumaric acid

Antioxidants

E300	Ascorbic acid
E301	Sodium ascorbate
E302	Calcium ascorbate
E303	Potassium ascorbate
E304	(i) Ascorbyl palmitate
	(ii) Ascorbyl stearate
E306	Tocopherol-rich extract
E307	Alpha-tocopherol
E308	Gamma-tocopherol
E309	Delta-tocopherol
E310 [A]	Propyl gallate
E311 [A]	Octyl gallate
E312 [A]	Dodecyl gallate
E315	Erythorbic acid
E316	Sodium erythorbate
E317	Erythorbin acid
E318	Sodium erythorbin
E319	Butylhydroxinon
E320	Butylated hydroxyanisole (BHA)
E321 [A]	Butylated hydroxytoluene (BHT)

Emulsifiers

E322	Lecithins
E325	Sodium lactate
E326	Potassium lactate
E327	Calcium lactate
E329	Magnesium lactate

E330	Citric acid
E331	(i) Monosodium citrate
	(ii) Disodium citrate
	(iii) Trisodium citrate
E332	Potassium citrates
	(i) Monopotassium citrate
	(ii) Tripotassium citrate
E333	(i) Monocalcium citrate
	(ii) Dicalcium citrate
	(iii) Tricalcium citrate
E334	Tartaric acid
E335	(i) Monosodium tartrate
	(ii) Disodium tartrate
E336	(i) Monopotassium tartrate
	(ii) Dipotassium tartrate
E337	Sodium potassium tartrate
E338	Phosphoric acid
E339	(i) Monosodium phosphate
	(ii) Disodium phosphate
	(iii) Trisodium phosphate
E340	(i) Monopotassium phosphate
	(ii) Dipotassium phosphate
	(iii) Tripotassium phosphate
E341	(i) Monocalcium phosphate
	(ii) Dicalcium phosphate
	(iii) Tricalcium phosphate
E343 [U]	(i) Monomagnesium phosphate
	(ii) Dimagnesium phosphate
E350	(i) Sodium malate
	(ii) Sodium hydrogen malate
E351	Potassium malate
E352	(i) Calcium malate
	(ii) Calcium hydrogen malate
E353	Metatartaric acid
E354	Calcium tartrate

Acidity Regulators

E355	Adipic acid
E356	Sodium adipate
E357	Potassium adipate
E363	Succinic acid
E365	Sodium fumarate

E366	Potassium fumarate
E367	Calcium fumarate
E370	1,4-Heptonolactone
E375 [A]	Nicotinic acid, niacin, nicotinamide
E380	Triammonium citrate
E381	Ammonium ferric citrate
E385	Calcium disodium ethylene diamine tetra-acetate (Calcium disodium EDTA)

Thickeners/Stabilizers/Emulsifiers

E400	Alginic acid
E401	Sodium alginate
E402	Potassium alginate
E403	Ammonium alginate
E404	Calcium alginate
E405	Propan-1,2-diol alginate
E406	Agar
E407 [A]	Carrageenan
E407a	Processed eucheuma seaweed
E410	Locust bean gum
E412	Guar gum
E413 [A]	Tragacanth
E414 [A]	Acacia gum (gum arabic)
E415	Xanthan gum
E416 [A]	Karaya gum
E417	Tara gum
E418	Gellan gum
E420	(i) Sorbitol
	(ii) Sorbitol syrup
E421	Mannitol
E422	Glycerol
E425	(i) Konjac gum
	(ii) Konjac glucomannane
E426 [U]	Soybean hemicellulose
E430	Polyoxyethylene (8) stearate
E431	Polyoxyethylene (40) stearate
E432	Polyoxyethylene sorbitan monolaurate (polysorbate 20)
E433	Polyoxyethylene sorbitan monooleate (polysorbate 80)
E434	Polyoxyethylene sorbitan monopalmitate (polysorbate 40)
E435	Polyoxyethylene sorbitan monostearate (polysorbate 60)
E436	Polyoxyethylene sorbitan tristearate (polysorbate 65)
E440	(i) Pectin
	(ii) Amidated pectin

E442	Ammonium phosphatides
E444	Sucrose acetate isobutyrate
E445	Glycerol esters of wood rosins
E450	(i) Disodium diphosphate
	(ii) Trisodium diphosphate
	(iii) Tetrasodium diphosphate
	(iv) Dipotassium diphosphate
	(v) Tetrapotassium diphosphate
	(vi) Dicalcium diphosphate
	(vii) Calcium dihydrogen diphosphate
E451	(i) Pentasodium triphosphate
	(ii) Pentapotassium triphosphate
E452	(i) Sodium polyphosphates
	(ii) Potassium polyphosphates
	(iii) Sodium calcium polyphosphate
(iv)	Calcium polyphosphates
E459	Beta-cyclodextrine
E460	(i) Microcrystalline cellulose
	(ii) Powdered cellulose
E461	Methyl cellulose
E462 [U]	Ethyl cellulose
E463	Hydroxypropyl cellulose
E464	Hydroxypropyl methyl cellulose
E465	Ethyl methyl cellulose
E466	Carboxy methyl cellulose, sodium carboxy methyl cellulose
E467 [U]	Ethyl hydroxyethyl cellulose
E468	Crosslinked sodium carboxymethyl cellulose
E469	Enzymically hydrolysed carboxy methyl cellulose
E470a	Calcium, potassium and sodium salts of fatty acids
E470b	Magnesium salts of fatty acids
E471	Mono- and diglycerides of fatty acids
E472a	Acetic acid esters of mono- and diglycerides of fatty acids
E472b	Lactic acid esters of mono- and diglycerides of fatty acids
E472c	Citric acid esters of mono- and diglycerides of fatty acids
E472d	Tartaric acid esters of mono- and diglycerides of fatty acids
E472e	Mono- and diacetyl tartaric acid esters of mono- and diglycerides of fatty acids
E472f	Mixed acetic and tartaric acid esters of mono- and diglycerides of fatty acids
E473	Sucrose esters of fatty acids
E474	Sucroglycerides
E475	Polyglycerol esters of fatty acids

E476	Polyglycerol polyricinoleate
E477	Propane-1,2-diol esters of fatty acids
E479b	Thermally oxidized soya bean oil interacted with mono- and diglycerides of fatty acids
E481	Sodium stearoyl-2-lactylate
E482	Calcium stearoyl-2-lactylate
E483	Stearyl tartrate
E491	Sorbitan monostearate
E492	Sorbitan tristearate
E493	Sorbitan monolaurate
E494	Sorbitan monooleate
E495	Sorbitan monopalmitate

Acidity Regulators/Improving Agents/Firming Agents

E500	(i) Sodium carbonate
	(ii) Sodium hydrogen carbonate
	(iii) Sodium sesquicarbonate
E501	(i) Potassium carbonate
	(ii) Potassium hydrogen carbonate
E503	(i) Ammonium carbonate
	(ii) Ammonium hydrogen carbonate
E504	(i) Magnesium carbonate
	(ii) Magnesium hydroxide carbonate
	(Magnesium hydrogen carbonate)
E507	Hydrochloric acid
E508	Potassium chloride
E509	Calcium chloride
E511	Magnesium chloride
E512	Stannous chloride
E513	Sulphuric acid
E514	(i) Sodium sulphate
	(ii) Sodium hydrogen sulphate
E515	(i) Potassium sulphate
	(ii) Potassium hydrogen sulphate
E516	Calcium sulphate
E517	Ammonium sulphate
E518	Magnesium sulphate (Epsom salts)
E519	Copper sulphate
E520	Aluminium sulphate
E521	Aluminium sodium sulphate
E522	Aluminium potassium sulphate
E523	Aluminium ammonium sulphate

E524	Sodium hydroxide
E525	Potassium hydroxide
E526	Calcium hydroxide
E527	Ammonium hydroxide
E528	Magnesium hydroxide
E529	Calcium oxide
E530	Magnesium oxide
E535	Sodium ferrocyanide
E536	Potassium ferrocyanide
E538	Calcium ferrocyanide
E541	Sodium aluminium phosphate, acidic
E542	Bone phosphate
E543	Calcium sodium polyphosphate
E544	Calcium polyphosphate
E545	Ammonium polyphosphate
E550	Sodium silicate
E551	Silicon dioxide
E552	Calcium silicate
E553a	(i) Magnesium silicate
	(ii) Magnesium trisilicate
E553b [A]	Talc
E554	Sodium aluminium silicate
E555	Potassium aluminium silicate
E556	Calcium aluminium silicate
E558	Bentonite
E559	Aluminium silicate (Kaolin)
E570	Fatty acids
E572	Magnesium stearate, calcium stearate

Acidity Regulators/Sequestrants

E574	Gluconic acid
E575	Glucono-delta-lactone
E576	Sodium gluconate
E577	Potassium gluconate
E578	Calcium gluconate

Colourings

E579	Ferrous gluconate
E585	Ferrous lactate
E586 [U]	4-hexylresorcinol

Flavour Enhancers

E620	Glutamic acid
E621	Monosodium glutamate
E622	Monopotassium glutamate
E623	Calcium diglutamate
E624	Monoammonium glutamate
E625	Magnesium diglutamate
E626	Guanylic acid
E627	Disodium guanylate
E628	Dipotassium guanylate
E629	Calcium guanylate
E630	Inosinic acid
E631	Disodium inosinate
E632	Dipotassium inosinate
E633	Calcium inosinate
E634	Calcium 5'-ribonucleotides
E635	Disodium 5'-ribonucleotides
E636	Maltol
E637	Ethyl maltol
E640	Glycine and its sodium salt
E650	Zinc acetate

Anti-foaming/Anti-caking Agent

E900	Dimethyl polysiloxane

Glazing Agents

E901 [A]	Beeswax, white and yellow
E902	Candelilla wax
E903 [A]	Carnauba wax
E904	Shellac
E905	Microcrystalline wax
E907	Crystalline wax (hydrogenated poly-1-decene)
E910	L-cysteine
E912	Montanic acid esters
E913	Lanolin
E914	Oxidized polyethylene wax
E915	Esters of Colophane

Improving Agents/Preservatives

E920	L-cysteine hydrochloride
E921	L-cysteine hydrochloride monohydrate
E924	Potassium bromate

E925	Chlorine
E926	Chlorine dioxide
E927	Azodicarbonamide

Propellants/Packaging Gases

E938	Argon
E939	Helium
E941	Nitrogen
E942	Nitrous oxide
E943a	Butane
E943b	Isobutane
E944	Propane
E948	Oxygen
E949	Hydrogen

Sweeteners

E950	Acesulfame K
E951	Aspartame
E952	Cyclamic acid and its Na and Ca salts
E953	Isomalt
E954	Saccharin and its Na, K and Ca salts
E955	Sucralose
E957	Thaumatin
E959	Neohesperidine DC
E962	Salt of aspartame (acesulfame)
E965	(i) Maltitol
	(ii) Maltitol syrup
E966	Lactitol
E967	Xylitol
E968 [U]	Erythritol

Thickening Agents/Stabilizers/Foaming Agents

E999	Quillaia extract
E1103	Invertase
E1105	Lysozyme
E1200	Polydextrose
E1201	Polyvinylpyrrolidone
E1202	Polyvinylpolypyrrolidone
E1400	Dextrin
E1401	Modified starch
E1402	Alkaline modified starch
E1403	Bleached starch

E1404	Oxidized starch
E1410	Monostarch phosphate
E1412	Distarch phosphate
E1413	Phosphated distarch phosphate
E1414	Acetylated distarch phosphate
E1420	Acetylated starch
E1421	Acetylated starch, mono starch acetate
E1422	Acetylated distarch adipate
E1430	Distarch glycerine
E1440	Hydroxy propyl starch
E1441	Hydroxy propyl distarch glycerine
E1442	Hydroxy propyl distarch phosphate
E1450	Starch sodium octenyl succinate
E1451	Acetylated oxidized starch

Humectant/Foam Stabilizer

E1505	Triethyl citrate
E1510	Ethanon
E1517	Glyceryl diacetate (diacetin)
E1518	Glyceryl triacetate (triacetin)
E1519	Benzyl alcohol
E1520	Propan-1,2-diol (propylene glycol)

Appendix B: Useful Contacts

Prebiotic/Probiotic Products

BioCare Limited
Professional Healthcare Specialists
Lakeside, 180 Lifford Lane, Kings Norton
Birmingham B30 3NU
Tel: 0121 433 3727 (Sales orders and general enquiries)
Tel: 0121 433 8702 (Technical Support)
e-mail: biocare@biocare.co.uk.
www.biocare.co.uk

Cow & Gate
Whitehorse Business Park
Trowbridge, Wiltshire BA14 0XQ
Tel: 08457 623623 (Careline)

Yakult UK Ltd
1216 Telford Way
Westway Estate
Acton, London W3 7XS
Tel: 020 8740 4111
www.yakult.co.uk

Charities/Campaign Groups
Action Against Allergy
PO Box 278, Twickenham TW1 4QQ
Tel: 020 8892 2711
www.actionagainstallergy.co.uk

CORE
(the new name for Digestive Disorders Foundation)
3 St Andrews Place
London NW1 4LB
www.corecharity.org.uk

IBS Network
Northern General Hospital
Sheffield S5 7AU
www.ibsnetwork.org.uk

Bibliography

Aggarwal, A, Cutts, T F, Abell, T L, et al. 'Predominant symptoms in irritable bowel syndrome correlate with specific autonomic nervous system abnormalities.' *Gastroenterology (1994);106:94550*

Barefoot, S F, Klaenhammer, T R. 'Detection and activity of Lactacin B, a bacvetiocin produced by *Lactobacillus* acidophilus.' *Applied Environmental Microbiology (1983);45:180815*

Bomba, A, Nemcova, R. 'Improvement of the probiotic effect of micro-organisms by their combination with maltodextrins, fructo-oligosaccharides and polyunsaturated fatty acids.' *British Journal of Nutrition (2002); 88:S95S99*

Bown, D. *The Royal Horticultural Society Encyclopedia of Herbs* (London: Dorling Kindersley, 1997)

Christensen, J. 'The enteric nervous system', in *An Illustrated Guide to Gastrointestinal Motility* (Chichester: John Wiley, 1998)

De Simone, C, Veseley, R, Bianchi, S B, et al. 'The role of probiotics in the modulation of the immune system in man and animals.' *International Journal of Immunotherapy* (1993);9:2328

De Vrese, M, Stegelmann, A, et al. 'Probiotics – compensation for lactase insufficiency.' *American Journal of Clinical Nutrition* (2001);73:421s29s

Dickhaus, B, Firooz, N, Stain, J, et al. 'Psychological stress increases visceral sensitivity in patients with irritable bowel syndrome (IBS) but not controls.' *Gastroenterology (2001);120:A-67*

Edwards, C A, Parrett, A M. 'Intestinal flora during the first months of life: new perspectives.' *British Journal of Nutrition* (2002);88: S11S18

Fung, D Y C, Ceylan, E, et al. 'Cinnamon is lethal weapon against E. coli 0157:H7.' *Innovations in Food Technology* (1999); p.18

Gibson, G R, Fooks, L J. 'Probiotics as modulators of the gut flora.' *British Journal of Nutrition* (2002);88:S39S49

Gibson, G R, Roberfroid, M. 'Dietary modulation of the human colonic microbiota: introducing the concept of prebiotics.' *Journal of Nutrition* (1995);125:140112

Harvey, R F, Mauad, E C, Brown, A M. 'Prognosis in the irritable bowel syndrome: a five-year prospective study.' *Lancet* (1987);1:9635

Holford, P. *The Optimum Nutrition Bible* (London: Piatkus, 1997)

Jiang, T, Savaiano, D A. 'In vitro lactose fermentation by human colonic bacteria is modified by *Lactobacillus* acidophilus supplementation.' *Journal of Nutrition* (1997);127:148995

Jones, J, et al. 'British Society of Gastroenterology Guidelines for the Management of the Irritable Bowel Syndrome.' *Gut* (2000): 47 (Suppl. 2)

Kalliomäki, M, Isolauri, E. 'Role of intestinal flora in the development of allergy.' *Current Opinion in Allergy and Clinical Immunology* (2003);3:1520

Lee, Y-K, Puong, K-Y. 'Competition for adhesion between probiotics and human gastrointestinal pathogens in the presence of carbohydrate.' *British Journal of Nutrition* (2002);88:S101S108

Lembo, T, Munakata, J, Mertz, H, et al. 'Evidence for hypersensitivity of lumbar splanchnic afferents in irritable bowel syndrome.' *Gastroenterology* (1994);107:168696

Madden, J A J, Hunter, J O. 'A review of the role of the gut microflora in irritable bowel syndrome and the effects of probiotics.' *British Journal of Nutrition* (2002);88:S67S72

Marin, M L, Lee, J H, et al. 'Differential cytokine production in clonal macrophage and T-cell lines cultured in bifidobacteria.' *Journal of Dairy Science* (1996)

Martineau, P, Seksik, P, Jian, R. 'Probiotics and intestinal health: a clinical perspective.' *British Journal of Nutrition* (2002);88:S51S57

Newcomer, A D, Park, H S, O'Brian, P C, et al. 'Response of patients with irritable bowel syndrome and lactase deficiency using unfermented acidophilus milk.' *American Journal of Clinical Nutrition* (1983); 38:25763

Pessi, T, Suttas, Y, et al. 'Antiproliferative effects of homogenates derived from five strains of candidate probiotic bacteria.' *Applied and Environmental Microbiology* (1999);65:472528

Plummer, S, Weaver, M, et al. '*Clostridium difficile* pilot study: effects of probiotic supplementation on the incidence of C. difficile diarrhoea.' *International Micobiology* (2004);7:5962

Rodriguez, L A G, Ruigomez, A. 'Increased risk of irritable bowel syndrome after bacterial gastroenteritis: cohort study.' *British Medical Journal* (1999);318: 56566

Sanders, M E. 'Considerations for use of probiotic bacteria to modulate human health.' *Journal of Nutrition* (2000);130:384s90s

Scarpignato, C, Rampal, P. 'Prevention and treatment of traveller's diarrhoea: a clinical pharmacological approach.' *Chemotherapy* 1995 ; 41:4881

Stanton, C, Gardiner, G, et al. 'Market potential for probiotics.' *American Journal of Clinical Nutrition* (2001);73:476s83s

Svendsen, J H, Munck, L K, Anderson, J R. 'Irritable bowel syndrome: prognosis and diagnostic safety. A 5-year follow-up study.' *Scandinavian Journal of Gastroenterology* (1985);20:41518

Szajewska, H, Mrukowicz, J Z. 'Probiotics in the treatment and prevention of acute infectious diarrhoea in infants and children: a systematic review of published randomised, double-blind, placebo-controlled trials.' *Journal of Pediatric Gastroenterology and Nutrition* (2001);33:S17S25

Thornley, J P, Brough, J, Wright, T, Neal, K R, Jenkins, D, Spiller, R C. 'Bacterial toxins influence long term bowel dysfunction following *Campylobacter* enteritis, program and abstracts of Digestive Disease Week.' May 2124 (2000); San Diego, California; Abstract 3841

Van Loo, J, Couseement, P, et al. 'On the presence of inulin and oligofructose as natural ingredients in the Western diet.' *Critical Reviews in Food Science and Nutrition* (1995);35(6):52552

Whitehead, W E, Crowell, M D, Robinson, J C, et al. 'Effects of stressful life events on bowel symptoms: subjects with irritable bowel syndrome compared to subjects without bowel dysfunction.' *Gut* (1992);33:82530

Wildwood, C. *The Encyclopedia of Healing Plants* (London: Piatkus, 1998)

Wood, J D.'Physiology of the enteric nervous system', in L R Johnson (ed.), *Physiology of the Gastrointestinal Tract* (NewYork: Raven, 1994):42382

Index to Recipes

HOW TO COPE SUCCESSFULLY WITH

IRRITABLE BOWEL SYNDROME

Richard Emerson

Irritable Bowel Syndrome is a complex problem with both physical and psychological symptoms. The aim of this book is to set out clearly and concisely these symptoms and the various treatments now available – conventional, complementary and alternative. Ths should enable sufferers to improve their lifestyle and either cure or manage their Irritable Bowel Syndrome.

ISBN: 1-903784-06-9

128p

HOW TO COPE SUCCESSFULLY WITH

COLITIS

Dr Tom Smith

We know a lot about the changes that occur in the bowel of people with colitis and how to return them to normal. It should be only a matter of time before we know *why* these changes happen. Colitis means 'inflammation of the large bowel' (the colon), inflammation takes several forms and doctors have different views from the general public on what constitutes colitis. Most of this book is devoted to ulcerative colitis and Crohn's, with chapters on how to distinguish these inflammatory bowel diseases from irritable bowel, diverticular disease and colon cancer.

ISBN: 1-903784-12-3

128pp

HOW TO COPE SUCCESSFULLY WITH

CROHN'S DISEASE

Dr Tom Smith

Although on Crohn's disease, this book compares the similarities and differences to ulcerative colitis. Dr Smith describes how modern medicine is used to relieve and prevent serious complications. He explains how the normal bowel works, how it can go wrong and why it can produce the three main symptoms of diarrhoea, bleeding and mucus. This book describes the tests, investigations, and the diagnosis of the illness. It is not just the illness but how much of the bowel is infected that affects the treatment and how quickly and completely recovery is made. Other bowel problems that mimic Crohn's are described.

ISBN: 1 903784 16 6   112pp

HOW TO COPE SUCCESSFULLY WITH

DIVERTICULITIS

Dr Joan McClelland

Diverticulitis is a Cinderella disorder. It is very common, can be dangerous and there are rapidly increasing numbers of sufferers. We stand a more than 50 per cent chance of suffering from diverticulitis before we reach the age of 60. Dr Joan McClelland describes in her easily accessible style the symptoms, different types of diverticulitis, complications and various treatments including alternative and herbal remedies. This book also covers the psychological aspects of diverticulitis and the benefits of exercise and diet.

ISBN: 1-903784-00-X   128pp

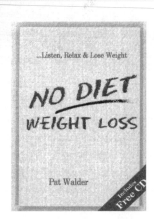

NO DIET
WEIGHT LOSS

Pat Walder

- Have you tried of an endless variety of diets?
- Do you find you lose some weight, then put it all back on again – plus a little more?
- Do you envy those people who can eat whatever they like and never put on weight?
- If you answered yes to any, or all, of the above questions, then what is contained within the pages **No Diet Weight Loss** will solve all your problems. This is a radical new way of achieving your perfect body weight and maintaining that weight PERMANENTLY – without diets, pills, potions or excessive exercise.

Dr Tom Smith said about this book:-

'This book is full of common sense and good advice on how to change one's life permanently to overcome all the habits that produce obesity. I will certainly recommend it to my patients. It gives people an excellent insight into themselves and how they have become overweight. It gives rational and sound advice on how to change their attitudes and lifestyle, not just so that they can be thinner, but happier with themselves, too. And it does this in a style that is easy to read, with humour and sympathy. An excellent book for everyone involved in obesity – and nowadays that means more than half of the adult population. I wish I had written it myself.'

ISBN 1-903784-10-7   88pp + CD